TO NOT
WEAR
BLACK

FIND YOUR STYLE, CREATE YOUR
FOREVER WARDROBE

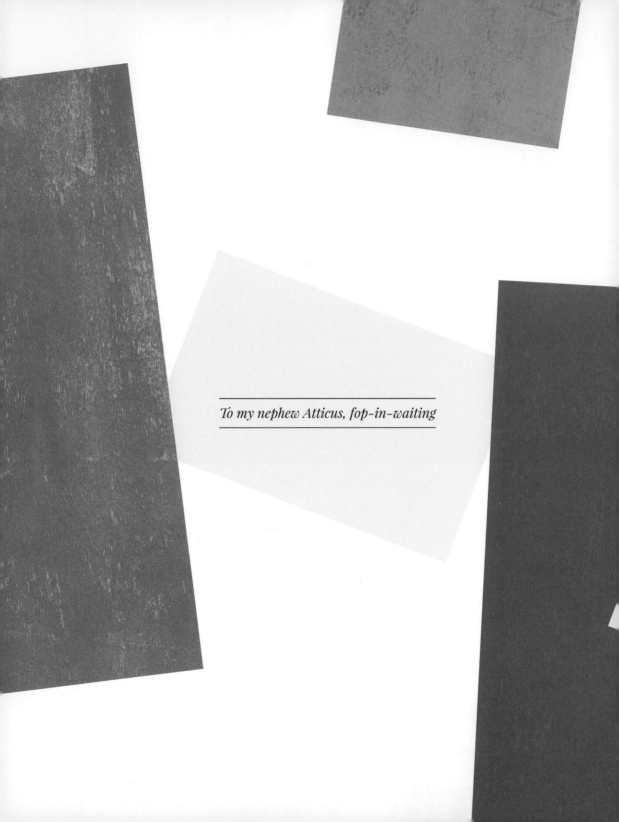

To my nephew Atticus, fop-in-waiting

HOW TO NOT WEAR BLACK

FIND YOUR STYLE, CREATE YOUR FOREVER WARDROBE

ANNA MURPHY

CONTENTS

Foreword

TORY BURCH

When I was five-years-old, I wanted to paint my bedroom mandarin orange. My mother, quite shrewdly, thought it would be a little much and we compromised on Kelly green.

I love color. I have for as long as I can remember. For me, color is tied to memory—burnt red reminds me of the clay tennis court where my mother taught me to play; earthy green brings back the feeling of summiting Machu Picchu with my boys a few years ago; and when I see pale pink, I think of the button-downs my dad wore while riding his tractor around our farm in Valley Forge.

My childhood was very colorful, in every sense of the word. We lived on a farm in the middle of nowhere, but on any given day the house was full of family and friends: artists, musicians, interior designers, writers .... Some would stay for dinner, some for weeks, some for years. You never knew, but it was always an adventure. My parents' door was always open.

My parents were both insatiably curious, drawn to colorful people and experiences. They were adventurers who saw the world together. Every summer they would board a big steamer ship, and

6

set sail for Greece, Morocco, or India, spending six weeks exploring different countries. They would come back from their trips with the most incredible objects—exotic textiles, curiosities, and hundreds of photographs. Each had a story. As soon as I was old enough I began traveling on my own, and I've essentially never stopped.

The vibrancy of my upbringing and my travels have shaped the way I see the world and, by extension, the way I design. When we start to design a new collection, we pull together inspiration images, photographs, swatches—but the overall story always starts with color. I'm drawn to mixing colors in unexpected ways.

Personal style is such an elusive concept, but at its core it's self-expression—an act of self-expression we all participate in every day. What I hope to express to the world is living life in full color with character, beauty, and confidence. It is my guiding principle and informs all that I do. Style is about so much more than what you wear—it's how you carry yourself, how you treat other people, your confidence, your essence, and in the end, your impact on others.

That said, telegraphing that essence can be tricky. No one is a better guide than Anna, who understands the intrinsically empowering effect clothes can have. Like Anna, my dressing philosophy

Style is about so much more than what you wear—it's how you carry yourself, how you treat other people ...

7

has always been to wear what makes you feel good and enhances your individuality. I am a self-admitted tomboy—growing up with three brothers will do that—and we have played with that masculine-feminine duality in all our collections. In high school, I used fashion to express myself. I was a frequent dress code violator, from personalizing my uniform with sewn patches to wearing colorful boxers under my kilt. The demerits were well worth it.

Clothes should, ultimately, function to make you feel like the best—and most authentic—version of yourself. They should empower you and give you the confidence to live your life in full color. Even if that means inspiring you to paint your bedroom mandarin orange …

Tory Burch

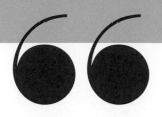

If you have the power to control how people see and interpret you, why not use it?

9

— RUPAUL

Introduction

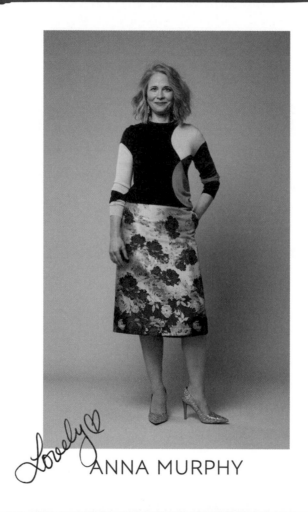

lovely♥

ANNA MURPHY

Fashion can be your friend, your ally; a source of joy, a form of empowerment. Clothes can be a way to express yourself; more than that, to discover yourself. But it can be hard to find your way to that friendship. Often clothes can seem like hard work. Sometimes they can seem like the enemy. That's why so many of us take the apparently easy route. We hide in plain sight in head-to-toe black. Or we give up altogether, and wear clothes that we've had for years, clothes that may or may not have suited us once upon a time, but are certainly no longer on our side. Neither approach represents being—living—your best self. And neither, in actuality, represents the easy route. Dressing you—not someone else's idea of you—will change your life for the better.

This book is a practical guide on how to do that; how to transcend the boring, without ever descending into fashion victim. It's about how to appear contemporary without seeming try-hard. And how to find those eternally existence-enhancing items of clothing that will change the way you look and feel, and that will be with you if not quite in perpetuity, then certainly for the next few chapters of your story. The forever wardrobe is not an impossible notion. And I am here to help you track it down.

How to nail your personal style once and for all? How to seek out the clothes that don't just work for you but that augment you, for life

The forever wardrobe is not an impossible notion. And I am here to help you track it down.

almost everlasting? It is not about abandoning what already serves you, but learning how to amp it up.

Which is why this book's title, *How to Not Wear Black*, isn't quite the full story. I am not saying don't wear this most practical of shades. Indeed, I will be suggesting more interesting ways to buy and wear this very hue. What I am saying is don't *only* wear black.

I wear black regularly, but always leavened with color, pattern, or embellishment. And still, as I grow older I find myself wearing less and less of it. Why? Because I relish ever more the power we women have at our fingertips by way of fashion. Yes, it is a power.

The designer Miuccia Prada once told me that she feels saddened by her female friends who, especially as they age, "hide because they don't want to express themselves through clothes, reject the feminine point of view." Even she understands the appeal of "giving up the problem" which is fashion. Even she, she said, laughing, sometimes likes to dress "boring bad." But she feels more strongly that she wants to preserve, to cherish "the feminine part of my life." And she draws an explicit link between what you wear and how you feel, how you think. Style, she continued, is about "fitting your brain with what you are wearing so that it makes sense to you." Don't you want to cherish your femininity? Don't you want your clothes to make sense to you? More than that, to make sense of you? "I think fashion has to support us," is how Christiane Arp, the editor of German *Vogue*, put it to me. "We have to wear clothes. The clothes should never wear us."

So many women I meet in my role as Fashion Director at *The Times of London* tell me that they feel fashion tries to trip them up.

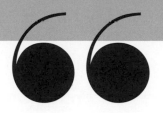

You will always be in fashion if you are true to yourself, and only if you are true to yourself.

—MAYA ANGELOU

They tell me that they have no idea about what to wear. Or that they did once upon a time, but that they have lost their way. Or, they tell me that they have ideas, but are worried about what others—a husband, a daughter, or generic "other people"—might think. They tell me they can't spend x; they don't deserve y.

They tell me, above all, that they love fashion, but that they also hate it. It always makes me think of Elena Ferrante's Neapolitan Novels, and her portrayal of an intense relationship between two women, Elena and Lila, that is a queasy kind of lovesickness, up and down, around and around. Too many of us are Elena to fashion's Lila, or is it the other way around?

This is partly the fault of the industry, endlessly encouraging us to buy more rather than to buy better; making us think that looking good is about following trends, rather than finding what works for each of us as individuals. But I believe it is also about bigger stuff than clothes. Fashion always is.

Some people—usually men—might consider clothes superficial fare. But fashion does matter. The dismissal of clothes by a to-date male-dominated culture as stuff and nonsense is, well, stuff and nonsense. The canny—men included—have long recognized that clothes equate with identity; more than that, with power. William Shakespeare wrote that "all the world's a stage" and that we are all "merely players." Costumes matter on a stage: they give clues as to who the "players" are, and what they want, where they might be going. Our everyday costumes do the same thing. Mark Twain— himself a fan of the all-white suit—wrote in his 1905 essay "The Czar's Soliloquy" that "There is no power without clothes. It is the

> **Dressing well is about self-worth. It's about believing in your place in the world; investing in it.**

power that governs the human race."

Dressing well is about self-worth. It's about believing in your place in the world; investing in it. It's about being bigger, bolder, and brighter—perhaps literally—than you might have been in the past. When you dress to impress, you stake your claim in the world to a voice, to a path, to a future. And you don't need money to do it. "I get more of a kick out of a ring that costs $4 than if my husband took me to Harry Winston," the nonagenarian fashion plate Iris Apfel once said to me.

Just to be clear, dressing to impress no longer means looking uptight. It might mean athleisure; it might mean jeans and a tee amped-up via a fabulous tuxedo jacket. Indeed, it might mean any number of different things. But what it definitely will mean are clothes that make you feel you; clothes that put a spring in your step, a smile on your face, and—most likely, by extension—a smile on the face of those around you. Wear your choices with confidence and you are already halfway there.

The good news is that fashion is less rule-bound than ever before. You can pick whatever suits you and the realities of your day-to-day. One example of what has changed is at the illustrious house of Dior. "Clothes for flower-like women" was what the famously dictatorial Christian Dior conjured up in the 1940s,

15

outfits that offered no room to maneuver, literally (you imagine trying to get onto a bus in the extravagantly skirted New Look of 1947) and metaphorically (if you weren't wearing the shape of the season you were an also-ran).

Now the illustrious house of Dior is headed up, for the first time, by a woman. And she is all about options. "In the real world you need different looks," says Maria Grazia Chiuri. "There are moments when you might feel more romantic, more rock-and-roll, more male, more sensual. Women change, even in the same day. I need to propose different ways to dress."

What a wonderful freedom: to choose what woman we want to be and to dress accordingly. Yet it can feel overwhelming. This book is here to help you realize that it needn't; that you, too, can find your way to what you love and, by extension, to who you are. We may sometimes envy men for the simplicity of their dress codes, but that simplicity also represents a kind of binding— so narrow is the bandwidth of what the average man can or can't wear.

The drag queen RuPaul is one notable male rule-breaker. But he believes that "drag" applies to all of us, that it's whatever we put on each morning. "And why not make it work for you? If you have the power to control how people see and interpret you, why not use it?" We women should celebrate our

What a wonderful freedom: to choose what woman we want to be and to dress accordingly.

sartorial latitude, much of it recent. Clothes can make our lives better. Read this book and I wager that yours will.

The late Maya Angelou spoke out over and over again about empowerment, telling women, black people, anyone who needed her encouragement, to "ask for what you want and be prepared to get it." When she spoke at events she would always dress to impress, perhaps in one of her favorite little black dresses with pearls. Black, yes—I told you it was still allowed—but transformed via statement jewelry. Not for her anymore the "plain ugly cut-down" she describes in her childhood autobiography I Know Why The Caged Bird Sings.

Angelou knew the power of words, and she knew the power of clothes, so I will let her have the final say: "Seek the fashion which truly fits and befits you. You will always be in fashion if you are true to yourself, and only if you are true to yourself."

Anna x

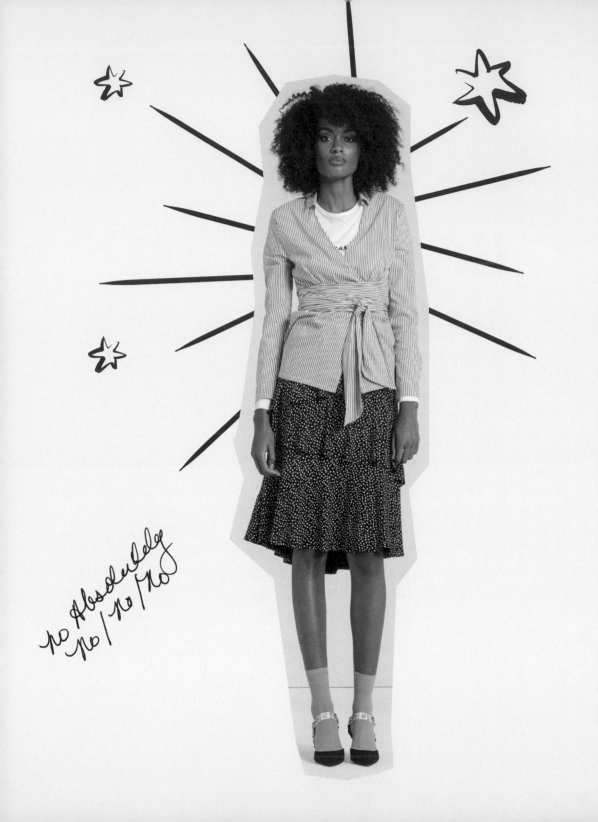

Bodymapping

FIGURING OUT YOUR
FIGURE, FINDING YOUR TRUE
FASHION FIXES

Most of us believe ourselves to be all too well acquainted with our body, and in particular its—our— supposed flaws. But are we really? And do we know how to dress that body to showcase it, to draw attention away from said flaws and toward what makes us fabulous?

What serves us best in every sphere of our life is self-knowledge, and most of us work hard to develop and expand it as we age. Yet when it comes to our body, and the clothes that will serve it best, we often remain ignorant.

Nail who you are physique-wise, and you'll be perfectly placed to find a style that suits you, and to curate a wardrobe that makes life easier and that makes you feel better in and of yourself. We all know about IQ, but what about "BIQ"? Develop your Body Intelligence Quotient and shopping, dressing—the whole once-fraught business of finding and then enjoying your personal style—will become child's play.

Why haven't we figured it out before? Because it's not easy to get your head around at first, and also because we aren't really told that it matters. Instead, trends are thrown at us, from the moment we first become aware that clothes represent choices; that fashion is a thing. Yet above all, as the ever quotable, ever wearable Coco Chanel once said, "Fashion is architecture. It is a matter of proportions." (You'll be hearing a lot from her in this book: she was as good at conjuring up sound bites as designing handbags.)

Coming to understand your proportions, the particular geometry of your body—and it is a kind of geometry—is a process. Many of us have at least one part we consider to be too large and therefore go about trying to disguise. Many of us have an idea that the relationship between, say, shoulder width and hip width impacts how we might look in a particular outfit. Many of us bandy around terms like "pear shape" and "apple shape" as if we were in a fruit shop. In fact, there are seven different body geometries (see p.27).

First, take a leaf out of the book of the famously sleek septuagenarian fashion designer Carolina Herrera. "The most

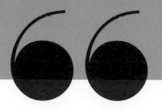

Fashion is architecture. It is a matter of proportions.

—COCO CHANEL

essential accessory a woman can have is a full-length mirror," she once told me. "Then you stand in front of it and ask, 'What do I need? What is wrong with me?'" If you don't have one at home already, buy one.

A mirror is key when shopping, too. If you want to find what really suits you, always shop in-store rather than online. Stand in front of the fitting room mirror. Is it you, or isn't it? Only part with money once you are sure it is. And beware of so-called vanity sizing, which can make a theoretically identical size entirely different from one brand to another. It doesn't matter what size it says on the label, just how it fits your body, how it makes you feel.

A mirror isn't just a matter of practicality. It's about seeing yourself in the most profound sense. "You either recognize yourself in the glass, or you don't," as Maria Grazia Chiuri, the creative director at the house of Dior, puts it. "Fashion is not only about clothes. There is more to it. For me, anyway."

One of the most important things to determine is whether you are at heart a formal or a casual person. Do you tend to overdress or to underdress? If you feel uncomfortable in a suit, it doesn't matter if you buy a great one; you will never put it on. If jeans always feel too sloppy for you, don't feel you have to wear them.

Grazia Chiuri told me how, when she was a child, her mother would dress her "in a way that didn't represent me, like a doll. I hated it. In Italy there is an obsession with looking 'nice,' and I wanted something different. In my mind a military jacket and jeans was me." At age 12, Grazia Chiuri set off unaccompanied to a flea market and, several buses later—"it felt like a big trip"—she found "that jacket, those jeans." When she got home, she looked in the mirror and saw herself for the first time. "I fought for the

It doesn't matter what size it says on the label, just how it fits your body, how it makes you feel.

22

clothes that were my clothes." We all need to find our clothes.

But what if you don't have a clear sense of what that possessive might apply to? We are bamboozled by choice now in a way that our grandmothers could never have imagined. It can be confusing enough to buy yogurt these days, never mind a dress.

BEYOND TRENDS

We are led to believe, in this consumer-driven society of ours, that fashion is about trends. We know we are supposed to keep an eye on them, but in doing so we fail to keep ourselves in focus. Trends are, as their name suggests, fly-by-night affairs. Your body is your lifelong partner. To learn its intricacies, and to develop a sense of what clothes suit it and what clothes don't, are the most important sartorial tools we can develop.

"Trends are not trendy," laughs the designer Roland Mouret. "Unless, of course, you want to be a trendy fashion person." Who wants to be that? Not me. Most of us want to put on a stress-free outfit in the morning and go about our day safe in the knowledge that we look our best. We want clothes we can forget about, in other words.

Is yellow "in"? Who cares if it doesn't suit you? How about boyfriend jeans? Ditto. As the red-carpet stylist Rebecca Corbin-Murray declares, "We should look for consistency rather than follow this idea, 'I need to make myself feel better, and pink is in this season, so I suddenly need to buy pink.' We need to stop going for that quick fix. Figure out what suits your body, what's your silhouette, then forget everything else."

Besides, the paradox is that although we think those quick fixes will make us happy—and in the short term, they might—in the long term they weigh us down. Corbin-Murray has recently done a wardrobe clear-out with one of her movie star clients. "She told me afterward, 'It is like a weight has lifted off me.'"

The style icons of the past didn't bother themselves with the hurly-burly of trends. Take Jackie Onassis, for example. "She knew exactly what was going to look good on her," recalls her friend

Herrera. "She knew exactly what she liked. She was never confused. If you look at old photographs of her, she still looks good for now."

"I wouldn't dream of following fashion," the famously idiosyncratic literary woman-about-town Edith Sitwell wrote in 1968. "How could one be a different person every three months?" Coco Chanel—told you—summed it up even better not once but twice. "Fashion changes but style endures." "Fashion is made to become unfashionable."

INTRODUCING THE PERMATREND

What it does make sense to pay some attention to is what I call permatrends. These are deeper shifts in the way people dress, and—precisely because they are so profound—there are very few of them. Permatrends may start off as apparently transient trends, but somehow they properly take hold, usually because there is something about them that chimes with the way we live and/or the way we want to be seen to live. Making them work for you— which can often be pulled off with just the subtlest of tweaks—is a way of looking effortlessly contemporary.

They tend to be broad brush strokes, a catch-all category rather than a one-off entity. Off-the-shoulder will never be a permatrend, for example. Big shoulders, on the other hand, defined the entire '80s and beyond, albeit in myriad different incarnations. They came of age at a time when women, for the first time in history, were beginning to be allowed to be—and therefore to look—strong. Men had long worn jackets with built-up shoulders to emphasize their alpha-maleness. Newly empowered in the workplace, a 1980s woman wanted—needed—to emphasize her alpha-maleness, too; to signpost that she could compete on a man's terms. Only later would there come a different kind of realization of strength: that you can be—and present as—100 percent woman, and still win.

Athleisure is another, more recent, permatrend that signifies something very different and yet still related. It's about casualness, sportiness, coolness: all those elements that are seen in the modern world as equating both to youth and to competency. It's one of the strange twists in which fashion specializes that a flourish of high-end, office-appropriate athleisure can these days suggest something akin to the power suit of yore. Mix a strong-shouldered jacket with satin track pants and you are pulling off permatrend point-scoring par excellence.

Because permatrends are catch-alls, they can usually be finessed to work for everyone. There is a pair of jeans out there for you, even if you haven't found them yet, and indeed I am here to help you find them. That said, if you are determined that there isn't, you can reference denim in other ways, perhaps by wearing the finest chambray shirt under tailoring, for example.

Similarly, athleisure doesn't have to be exclusively laid-back and teenage-looking, especially if you seek out classy fabrics and add-on embellishment. There are some wonderfully high-end, nay, chic takes on what was once reserved for the gym and the street. Even if you wear the neatest of iterations it will still give you a glow of youth.

But, to reiterate, permatrends can also be ignored. Everything can be, apart from what works for your body, which is—ironically—what most of us ignore most of the time. So let's get a clearer idea of what that might be.

66 *Permatrend:*
Jeans
Leopard Print

25

> **There is a pair of jeans out there for you, even if you haven't found them yet, and indeed I am here to help you find them.**

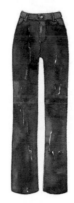

THE SEVEN SHAPES

As I said, there are seven main shapes: the neat hourglass, the full hourglass, the triangle, the inverted triangle, the column, the rectangle, and the rounded.

Many of us, myself included, will be a combination of two shapes. While hourglass shapes tend not to coexist—an hourglass is an hourglass—the others can and do. I, for example, am both a triangle—with full hips and thighs—and an inverted triangle, with square, broad shoulders and (sigh) not much of a waist.

OPERATION HOURGLASS

Why does this matter? Because in order to look our best we should all be engaged in a what I call Operation Hourglass or, to be more precise, Operation Neat Hourglass. That is the most in-proportion look of all, and we can all come closer to presenting as such if we develop a few tricks. As with everything else in fashion there are no hard and fast rules, but there are some handy markers.

If you are an hourglass in the first place then obviously you have it easiest. You need to wear clothes that follow your lines, not hide them. If you are a full hourglass make sure to favor fabrics that won't add bulk.

In general, color, pattern, and embellishment are going to draw attention to the section of the body where they are worn. So if you are a triangle you want to keep the focus on your top half; if you are an inverted triangle, on the bottom.

Stripes can be a particularly useful tool. To elongate, use verticals. To amp up a small bust or narrow hips, go for horizontals. Diagonals can bamboozle the eye, and in so doing smooth and balance out-of-proportion elements. Frills and gathers—vertical, horizontal, diagonal—will all function in the same way, but will, of course, add literal volume, too, as will rows of buttons.

TO BELT OR NOT TO BELT?

Bear in mind that a belt is the ultimate horizontal line, spotlighting your waist, or lack thereof. Fashion folk love to exhort us all to belt ourselves a waist, but that only works if you've got an approximation of one in the first place, or can afford to add volume elsewhere in order to fake it to make it.

Even the largest hourglass will look great in a belt. The slimmest column figure, on the other hand—by definition unwaisted—will only be flattered by a belt if they amp things up at the shoulders

There are seven different body geometries, a number of which can exist in pairs, meaning that someone can be two things at once.

Inverted triangle: *a straight, square shoulder line; little definition between waist and hips; flat hips and bottom; and a lower half that appears smaller than the upper.*

Neat hourglass: *a defined waist, a defined bust, and a neat bottom and hips.*

Column: *narrow shoulders, a flat chest or small bust, and undefined waist, plus narrow hips and a flat bottom.*

Full hourglass: *a defined waist, a full bust, and a full bottom and hips.*

Rectangle: *straight up and down (like the column) but, as the nomenclature suggests, wider, with square shoulders.*

Triangle: *full hips and thighs, a defined waist, shoulders that are narrow and/or sloping, and a top half that overall appears smaller than the lower.*

Rounded: *a rounded shoulder line, fullness around the middle, and a flattish bottom.*

and/or hips. Even then they might be better served by a peplum jacket or a full skirt. If you are rounded or rectangular, don't even go there.

SKIM TO WIN

Never swamp a part of your body that you feel is too large. When in doubt, skim. A tapered pencil skirt, for example, can look great on someone with bigger hips, provided there's something on the top half that adds balancing emphasis to the shoulders. Trick the eye into thinking the big bits are smaller, the small bits bigger, and that the relationship between the two is proportional.

For a large bust, choose simple tops that are well cut, plus consider any of the following: wrap styles, narrow lapels, soft fabrics, scoop necks, under-bust seams or darts, or ruching. For a small bust, invest in a padded or molded bra that has been fitted by an expert, then make hay with detailing on your top: breast pockets, buttons, smocking, statement sleeves, or—if you have got the upper arms for it—spaghetti straps or strapless. V-necks work on almost everyone.

The hardest body shapes to dress tend to be the rectangular and the rounded. It's easy to make the mistake of thinking unwaisted styles will work best, but again you want to skim, not swamp. A dress or top that is fitted to below the bust, then flares into a subtle A-line will probably be a good bet. Always remember to take a look at yourself sideways as well as straight on to check that an outfit flatters there, too.

If you want to minimize a tummy you should look for semi-fitted styles that cleave to the top of the body, then again become looser—but not too loose—around the middle. When it comes to

Bear in mind that a belt is the ultimate horizontal line, spotlighting your waist, or lack thereof.

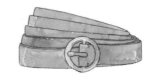

28

dresses, try an <u>empire line</u>, a <u>semi-fitted shift</u>, a <u>subtle A-line, or a</u> <u>coat dress</u>. Flat-fronted trousers are your friend, and so are prints and patterns, provided you factor in your frame size, see p.32. A longer cut of jacket can also work well.

Trick the eye into thinking the big bits are smaller, the small bits bigger, and that the relationship between the two is proportional.

*THE ULTIMATE WARDROBE ESSENTIAL

<u>Jackets.</u> You need one. The best bit of tailoring you can afford. There's not a woman in the front row who doesn't have at least one on repeat. To buy well and to wear it well, in a contemporary way (perhaps undone over a floral dress or paired with jeans and a tee), is a one-stop way to make yourself look current. The fashion pack favors a double-breasted style, but you need to buy what's right for your shape. Those two rows of buttons can be widening—the stripe affect again—so be careful if you have a medium or large bust or are a bigger size. (Though leaving it casually undone and wearing a more sculpted top underneath may be enough of a retool.) A very fitted style with visible seaming can do the trick if you are curvy. If you have a straight shape and a small bust you can try a boxy cut.

The <u>single-breasted approach is more universally flattering</u> but, again, if <u>you are curvy, go fitted, darted, and seamed.</u> And look for a <u>jacket length that works with the length of your torso and legs.</u> If you are short in the torso and long in the leg, search out a longer-line jacket. If you are long in the torso and short in the leg then a shorter jacket will probably suit you better.

THE FRAME GAME

Measure your wrists, then follow the chart on p.32 to ascertain whether you are a small, medium, or large frame, which refers to the size of your bones, and is unconnected to height or weight.

29

Pick patterns that chime with your frame, and accessories that do the same. Skinny shoes will make a big frame appear clumpy, clumpy shoes will make a skinny frame seem fly-away. A bold pattern will flatter a big frame, but dwarf a small one. Think middle, middle, middle for everything if yours is a medium frame.

Seek out the brands that work best for your frame and shape, as well as your aesthetic. Often, brands from a country where lots of women share your physique will serve you well. If you are petite, try French brands like Maje and Sandro, and Spanish brands like Zara. If you are tall, Scandinavian labels such as Cos, Ganni, and Arket—all popular with the front row—work well, as do J.Crew and Gap. Good brands for the curvy include Phase Eight and John Lewis's Modern Rarity, plus—if you are ready to invest— Vivienne Westwood and Issey Miyake's Pleats Please.

Shopping within one brand for a particular look is a great way to find pieces that work well together aesthetically. It is the job of people called merchandisers to make sure a collection functions as a whole: that's how they hope to tempt the consumer to buy more. Use this to your advantage. You will know you are getting it right, and it will also help you develop confidence that will enable you to mix and match brands with panache a little further down the line.

Then there's your frame shape to factor in, which is different from your frame size. Are you angular—all edges? Are you rounded and soft? Or are you a mix of the two, otherwise known as interjacent. You should be able to figure it out by looking in that mirror again. (See? Told you you would get your money's worth.)

You should go with fabrics that echo your lines, rather than oppose them. Sharp tailoring will look good on the angular, while soft lines will make them look more angular still. Soft lines will flatter the rounded. If you are interjacent you can pick and choose, plus you can play with different textures in a way that can be tricky for the other two.

Be realistic, too, about the fabrics that are going to work with your lifestyle. If you are a machine-washing kind of a girl—I know

Magic is a strong word. But a great jacket can deliver something close. It's a staple for every fashion professional I know because it can effortlessly change up any look. The latest tweak is to wear a mannish style open over a feminine skirt or dress. But the jacket can be your best friend for other reasons. Buy the best cut and the best kind of detailing for your shape and size and it will spotlight you in just the right way.

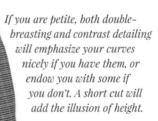

Single-breasted works on everyone, but is especially good if you are more broad. Change up predictable black or navy for a more interesting, yet still stealth hue like forest green.

If you are petite, both double-breasting and contrast detailing will emphasize your curves nicely if you have them, or endow you with some if you don't. A short cut will add the illusion of height.

FIGURING OUT YOUR FRAME SIZE			
Height	*Small framed*	*Medium framed*	*Large framed*
under 5'2"	wrist less than 5½in	wrist 5½in to 5¾in	wrist over 5¾in
5'2" to 5'5"	wrist less than 6in	wrist 6in to 6¼in	wrist over 6¼in
over 5'5"	wrist less than 6¼in	wrist 6¼in to 6½in	wrist over 6½in

I am—then buy as little as possible that is dry clean only. The
good news is that certain female-led brands are now specializing
in dresses and tailoring that looks to be dry clean but that can
actually be put in a cool wash. Bear in mind as well that many
brands stick dry-clean-only labels on silks and other delicates
that, in truth, can happily be put through a hand-wash cycle.

Once you understand your figure, and how its different
elements interact, you will get a better idea as to how the clothes
you wear interact, too. I am not going to pretend this stuff is easy,
although it will become second nature if you practice it. In the
meantime, there'll be some trial and error involved, of course.
But one good way to train your eye is to find a woman in the
public eye who has a similar body shape to you and whose style
you admire. Look and learn from how she dresses.

BE YOUR BEST BODY

Which brings me to you, the person wearing the clothes. The
body. Invest the time and energy it takes to find your way to
the best body you can, by which I don't mean the thinnest. It's
not about changing your shape. Indeed, that's another fallacy with
which we are indoctrinated: that if you just exercise hard enough
you will end up with thin thighs, a flat stomach, or whatever it is
we are supposed to covet.

I imagine you don't need to me to tell you that you are unlikely
to achieve so-called perfection. But what you can acquire is the
healthiest, strongest version of your own beautiful body. It doesn't

matter what size you are, as long as you are looking after your body as it deserves—as you deserve. The most important thing you will ever wear is your own flesh. That, more than any dress, any pair of jeans, will determine how you feel about yourself.

For me it has been yoga that has led me firstly to accept my shape, and then to commit to making it feel the very best I can. If that has also left me able to wear sleeveless tops—hurrah!—so much the better. But what I love is that I am stronger, more physically grounded in my mid-forties than in my mid-twenties. My body may not look as "good," but it feels better, and it looks pretty darn OK. It's an equation that has left me more at peace with my corporeal self than ever in my life before.

Find a woman in the public eye who has a similar body shape to you and whose style you admire. Look and learn from how she dresses.

It is not important what your thing is. It is only important that you have a thing. It might be yoga, pilates, or *chi gong*, all of which—from the women I know in their 60s and 70s who practice them—are brilliant disciplines for age-proofing your mind and body. It might be as simple as a brisk 40-minute walk every day, more than enough aerobic exercise according to many experts, plus some stretching and some work with light weights (which can be far more enjoyable than it sounds).

Strengthening and opening your back and chest in particular will improve your posture. And great posture will transform the way you look, making you stand like Grace Kelly, even in a sweatshirt and cargo pants.

FIND YOUR FOOD HAPPY PLACE

Then there's eating. So many of us are stuck in a dieting cycle, in a state of famine that is then inevitably followed by an out-of-control feast. We have lost touch with when we are genuinely

33

The towel test

Stand in front of that long mirror of yours and hold a bath towel by the two top corners of one of the shorter sides, the opposite side lightly touching the floor. Now lift the towel gradually upward, looking at your lower legs as they are revealed. There will be two points of elevation at which—hey, presto!—your legs look their prettiest. Those are the skirt lengths for you.

The expensive brands have always been well aware of the power of the long skirt, but the more affordable brands are finally—finally— waking up to it, too.

Never buy a skirt that's too short, but by all means buy too long, then get it altered.

hungry, and when we are satiated. Follow the true appetites of your body and you will end up your natural size, which may be precisely the size you are, or may be considerably smaller.

Bear in mind, too, that each body has its own issues. You may feel you have your crosses to bear, but so do other people who you might have thought have it easy. The flat-chested may dream of breasts, but as anyone with ample cleavage can testify, it's hard to find clothes that fit, and any kind of detailing, even something as apparently simple as a ribbed finish, can cause problems. I have always coveted smaller hips. But small hips can make the waist look larger. Make peace with what you have got. Better still, celebrate it.

TRICKS OF THE TRADE

Simplest of all is to showcase those bits of the body that are the most elegant on us all: our wrists and ankles. That's why cropped trousers tend to work so well, whatever your height. That's why a skirt length that cuts just below the fullest part of the calf, thus drawing attention to the ankles, is often the most flattering.

But—as I said—not always. Most of us have two points on the leg that work best for us, the second being higher up, and around the region of the knee—above it, below it or somewhere actually on the patella. Try the towel test (see left) to ascertain exactly which are the best lengths for you, and, if necessary, alter accordingly.

Indeed, that's the way to go generally. Alter, alter, alter. That's what stylists do. That's what the front row does. If you can't find something that fits, or—as is more often the case—you find something that fits in one area but is too small or large in another, buy the size that best fits your biggest part and get a tailor to adjust the rest. Finding and making friends with a professional tailor is almost as important as understanding and making friends with your body.

"I want women to look beautiful," Carolina Herrera once said. "I am in the beauty business, not the fashion business." And, of course, Coco Chanel had something to say on the matter, too. "Beauty comes when fashion succeeds." Dress to look your most beautiful, your most you. That's what matters.

36

No No No

There's a dress to flatter every figure.

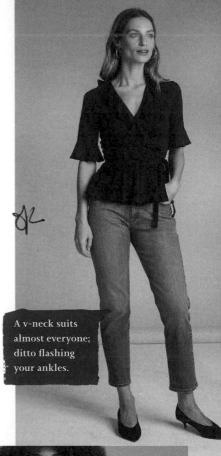

A v-neck suits almost everyone; ditto flashing your ankles.

A patterned lower half and a simple top will balance out an inverted triangle.

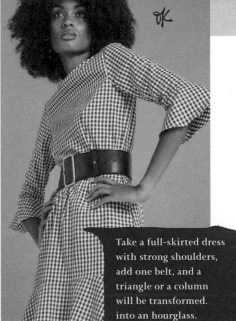

Take a full-skirted dress with strong shoulders, add one belt, and a triangle or a column will be transformed into an hourglass.

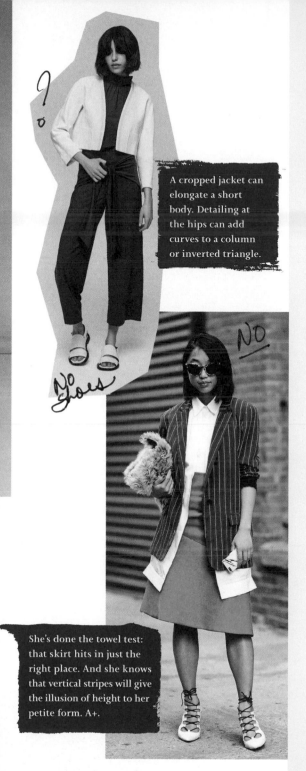

A cropped jacket can elongate a short body. Detailing at the hips can add curves to a column or inverted triangle.

NO Shoes

NO

She's done the towel test: that skirt hits in just the right place. And she knows that vertical stripes will give the illusion of height to her petite form. A+.

THE TOPOGRAPHY OF YOU

Learning how to navigate your body is the most important skill you can develop when it comes to finding your way with fashion, and turns buying and wearing clothes into a pleasure. We aren't taught this stuff when we are growing up, so at first it might not come easy. But it's like anything else in life: practice makes perfect. This chapter should have helped you identify your particular figure, and given some guidelines as to how best to dress it. Now head to a department store and start bodymapping for real. Try two different jacket lengths. See what they do for you. Two different dress shapes. At first it might seem overwhelming. In time it will become second nature.

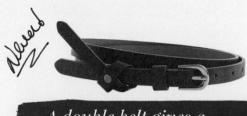

A double belt gives a contemporary feel.

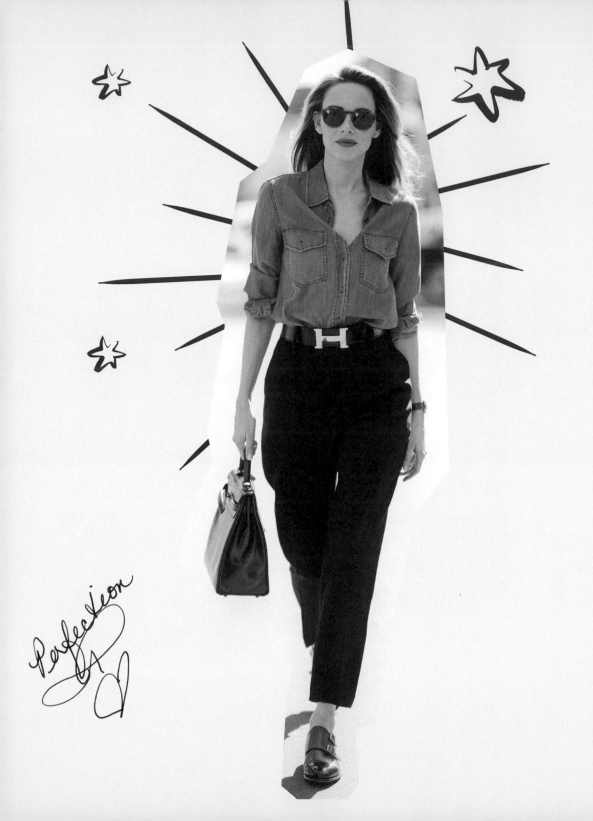

2

The Happy- Ever-After *Wardrobe*

WHAT TO GET RID OF, HOW TO DO IT

There is no greater joy than nailing your happy-ever-after wardrobe. This means ensuring that every item hanging in your closet is a Prince Charming; that there's not a fashion frog to be seen. How to make like fashion's own Sleeping Beauty? By finding what works for you, not following someone else's ideas on the matter.

It's easy to think that looking good is about being on-trend. That's the conclusion the fashion industry wants us to draw because that's what keeps us spending money. Oooh, it's all about blue. Oh no, actually you aren't anyone if you aren't in green this season. It has to be skinny jeans, or no, make that boyfriends. The pencil skirt is suddenly hot until it just as suddenly isn't, and it has to be the midi. ∫ all very true

Yet, tellingly, the very people who conjure up these trends—the designers themselves—tend to wear ensembles so plain, so unvarying, that they look as if they might be in the military, if the military were down with head-to-toe body-con and heels (Donatella Versace) or a high-collared shirt and leather driving gloves (Karl Lagerfeld).

And the people who then tell us about this stuff—journalists like me—also tend to be almost as focused with their own attire. Anna Wintour, the editor of American *Vogue*, wears the same shape of dress on repeat—full skirt, fitted top—and has been sporting identical Manolo nude kitten heels for eons.

WHY EDIT?

All of the above individuals have figured out their clothing happy place: what they feel most flatters their body and/or expresses their sense of self. And so they stick to it. They have found, in short, their personal style.

It's not only that. If you ask this breed of fashion professional why they limit themselves in this way, they will usually say—if they are being honest—that it's because they like not to have to think about what they wear each morning. This leaves them with a clear head for thinking about other things—in their case, what

40

"

It's always better to be underdressed.

—COCO CHANEL

other people might want to wear. Then they spend their day designing those clothes, or editing a magazine about them, or whatever.

To which I say, don't we all want that clear head? Don't we all have other things to think about than conjuring up a new look every day? If even Anna Wintour doesn't see fit to do it, then why should we? Don't we all, like her, want to know that our clothes are quietly getting on with the business of serving us, day in, day out; year in, year out? We, too, need to keep it simple. Less really is more. Or, as Coco Chanel once said, "It is always better to be underdressed."

If we want to add in a delicious complication or two later—in the form of some quirky footwear or jewelry—that's fine. But unless one has endless amounts of time, money, and a supremely honed style skill-set, the bare bones of one's wardrobe should be, well, considerably more bare than they probably are now. Most of us have far more in our closets than we actually wear. A recent survey estimated that people only wear about 20 percent of what they own. *20% 80% of the time*

"I hate trends," says red-carpet stylist Rebecca Corbin-Murray. "I feel like we've been locked in this game of trends for the longest time. More, more, more. Buy, buy, buy. A lot of people come to me with very little idea of what they like, what suits them. We're thrown trends all the time and mostly people just see what sticks, and then they have these bits and pieces, and don't know who they are, what their style is." It seems, like us, even movie stars have a wardrobe full of unrelated trends that don't work together, and that don't work for them.

> **Most of us have far more in our closets than we actually wear.**

THE 666 APPROACH

To find our own style mojo, we first need to get rid of those "bits and pieces" that are getting in the way, those items we don't currently wear, or that we wear but that don't suit us. I am not going to pretend that this isn't a hard process. But, though I say it myself, I think I have the modus operandi down pat.

I call it The 666 approach. Six piles and six questions make up stage one. Six months make up stage two. And though at times the process may – as the nomenclature suggests – feel positively devilish whilst in train, I hereby pledge that it will deliver you to wardrobe heaven in the end. So here we go…

STAGE ONE: 6 + 6

EVENING ONE: take everything out and sort it into six piles. (Do not—repeat, do not—fortify yourself with a glass of wine, medicinal as it may well seem at this point.) Those piles are:

1. Not worn for six months.
2. Used to fit but doesn't any more, and/or has become shabby (no kicking-about-the-house-only garb allowed).
3. Used to fit your lifestyle but doesn't any more.
4. Workwear.
5. Off-duty wear.
6. Occasionwear.

EVENING TWO: go through each of those piles, being as brutal as you can with the first three in particular. And, again, without even a soupçon of Chardonnay to help—or rather, hinder—the matter at hand. Try to remain detached and clear-headed throughout. Don't try too much on. Ask the following six questions about each item:

1. Does it fit me now?
2. Might it fit me in the next six months, no miracle required?
3. Do I look good when I wear it?
4. Do I feel good when I wear it? (In the double sense that it is both comfortable and flattering. When it comes to the latter, you need already to have bodymapped your way to having a clear sense of what does and doesn't work for your figure, as described in Chapter 1.)
5. Is it an unnecessary duplicate of another item that does the same job better?

6. Does it have sentimental value? (By which I mean genuine sentimental value. A bequest from Great Aunt Edith is valid, maybe. That this was your first ever pair of jeans and you haven't been able to fit into them since, is not.)

If the answer is not in the affirmative to at least four questions, get rid of it. Yes: you heard me. Depending on its quality and condition you might want to consider reselling it online, donating it to a thrift shop, or offering it to friends and family. Otherwise, take it to your nearest recycling bin.

Hang everything back in your closet, or put them back in your drawers. These days I prefer to have all my clothes out and available, rather than storing one season under the bed or in the attic. The seasons are becoming so variable, and central-heating can render you too hot in the winter, air-conditioning too cold in the summer.

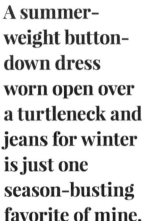

> **A summer-weight button-down dress worn open over a turtleneck and jeans for winter is just one season-busting favorite of mine.**

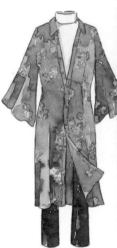

Then there's what I call new-generation layering (covered in detail in Chapter 7), which means that I am mixing-and-non-matching from largely the same wardrobe, be it January or June. A summer-weight button-down dress worn open over a turtleneck and jeans for winter is just one season-busting favorite of mine.

What's more, packing half your clothes away can prompt accidental duplicate purchasing, because the stores start pushing winter clothes when summer is in full swing, and vice versa. If you can see what you have, you aren't so likely to buy identical items.

And it's difficult to look after your clothes carefully when they're under the bed or in the attic compared to when they're hanging

SIX PILES

On the first evening, sort everything into six piles:

1. *Not worn for six months*
2. *Used to fit but doesn't any more, or has become shabby*
3. *Used to fit your lifestyle but doesn't any more*
4. *Workwear*
5. *Off-duty wear*
6. *Occasionwear*

SIX QUESTIONS

On the second evening, go through each of those piles.
Ask the following six questions about each item:

1. *Does it fit me now?*
2. *Might it fit me in the next six months, no miracle required?*
3. *Do I look good when I wear it?*
4. *Do I feel good when I wear it?*
5. *Is it an unnecessary duplicate of another item that does the same job better?*
6. *Does it have sentimental value?*

If the answer is not yes to at least four questions, get rid of it. Hang everything else back in your closet or return them to your drawers.

SIX MONTHS

For six months, every time you take something out of your wardrobe to wear, turn the hanger the other way around. By the end you will have incontrovertible evidence as to what you still have left that you don't wear.

Divide and rule

One change in my wardrobe organization has been to arrange by use and occasion (workwear, off-duty wear, etc.). I find this saves me time when getting dressed. It has also made it more straightforward to identify what's missing.

Because you will be missing things. Many of us—myself included—tend to repeat-buy what we already have rather than filling in the gaps. We don't focus enough on tracking down those workhorse separates that will connect the wardrobe dots for us. That's partly because these are the items that can be the most difficult to find, but I think it's also because they don't deliver the same shopping hit as something more showy.

I love a game-changer jacket, for example, and have no compunction investing in one that's gorgeous, but I didn't used to be so good at the pretty underlayer—blouse, silk tee, thin sweater—essential to enable said jacket to work its magic. Now I am always keeping my eyes peeled for that underlayer, and I buy more than one if I find a piece that really delivers.

in your closet. Once you have honed in on what's in your possession that is a fashion friend, not frenemy, you will want to hold on to it for as long as possible. Which means keeping it in good condition.

Finally, the onerous task of the seasonal switcheroo used to hang over me, and so would tend to get delayed until the relevant season was well under way. (Ski pants in summer? That's not what I mean by season-busting!) Save your efforts for turning your wardrobe overhaul into an annual, or at the very least biannual, event. Yes, really. You didn't think I was going to let you get off that lightly, did you?

Besides, I promise you will thank me. And you may even start to enjoy the editing process. The red-carpet stylist Elizabeth Saltzman—who works with Gwyneth Paltrow, among others— loves it. "I edit. That's what I do. My wardrobe at home is one rail. I have my uniform. And none of it is new. I don't understand the phenomenon of buying to throw it away." Why have three so-so black jackets when you can have one fabulous one? Buy less that's better. Keep it forever if it proves to be a true friend. And edit, edit, edit those frenemies. As Rebecca Corbin-Murray says, "Once you declutter it helps define who you are on a daily basis. It makes life so much easier."

Give a huge sigh of relief now that the first phase is over. And an even bigger one when you open your closet doors and drawers the next morning to the bliss of clothes you can actually see, clothes you can actually wear.

Have a couple of weeks' break from the whole fandango. Then, brace yourself for ...

STAGE TWO: THE FINAL 6

For six months, every time you take something out of your wardrobe to wear, turn the hanger the other way around. By the end you will have incontrovertible evidence as to what you still have left that you don't wear. And in the process you will, like as not, have dressed with more variety and imagination than you

47

normally do, wearing those things that you truly love but for whatever reason normally shy away from, for fear of losing them.

It's trickier to demarcate things so clearly when it comes to drawers and cabinets, but you can achieve similar if you have the means to compress what you have into half the space and gradually move things into the resulting empty drawers as and when you wear them. Once that same six-month time window closes, the rest—you guessed it—goes.

You are left with what actually works for you. And—trust me—there is nothing more freeing than to open a closet that presents solutions rather than problems. This is the point at which you can again address the gaps: look at what you are missing, what you need. Which is probably not whatever trend is being hawked en masse in the stores right now, but is instead the kind of classic pieces that have stood the test of time.

THE DOYENNE'S DOZEN

48 * A trench coat. A tuxedo suit. A cashmere sweater. A pair of loafers or ballet flats. Some classically cut jeans. A Breton top. A little black dress. Some white sneakers. A white or cream shirt or blouse. An olive utility jacket. A peacoat. If you had in your wardrobe nothing else but that doyenne's dozen—not one more, like a baker's, but one fewer; as I said, less is more—you would always look chic. You might not look exciting, but who needs to look exciting? Coco Chanel never looked exciting. Jackie O never looked exciting. Katharine Hepburn never looked exciting. They just looked their incredible best.

Most of the women who are known for their sense of style today are similarly focused. In some ways, they shop like the cliché of the 1950s man. Take Alexa Chung, for example. "Yes, that's me!" she laughed, when I once asked her if she recognized herself in that description. "I'm looking for things I have already, but maybe with small tweaks. When I shop I buy the checked shirt, the Breton top, the loafers. All the things I'm drawn to I've come to realize I had a version of as a child."

"

Once you declutter it helps define who you are on a daily basis. It makes life so much easier.

—REBECCA CORBIN-MURRAY

The doyenne's dozen

- ♡ TRENCH COAT
- ♡ TUXEDO SUIT
- ♡ CASHMERE SWEATER
- ♡ PAIR OF LOAFERS OR BALLET FLATS
- ♡ CLASSICALLY CUT JEANS
- ♡ BRETON TOP
- ♡ LITTLE BLACK DRESS
- ♡ WHITE SNEAKERS
- ♡ WHITE OR CREAM SHIRT OR BLOUSE
- ♡ OLIVE UTILITY JACKET
- ♡ PEACOAT

You don't need much, it just needs to be the best you can afford.

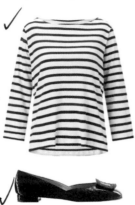
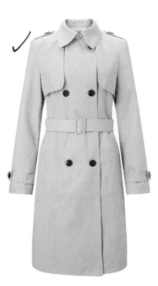

What I'd add

- ♡ FLORAL DRESS
- ♡ PATTERNED BLOUSE
- ♡ JUMPSUIT
- ♡ SHEARLING VEST
- ♡ BRIGHT BLAZER
- ♡ A COUPLE MORE CASHMERE SWEATERS
- ♡ PATTERNED FLOATY SKIRT
- ♡ CROPPED PANTS IN A NEUTRAL SHADE
- ♡ EMBELLISHED FLATS
- ♡ AN ARRAY OF EARRINGS AND LIPSTICKS

Or how about Christiane Arp, the neutral tailoring-garbed editor of German *Vogue?* "I do not believe in trends," she once told me. "I believe in good and bad fashion. I want you to have to ask what I am wearing, not to know." What I know about Arp is that she is always one of the most effortlessly dressed—most herself-looking—women on the front row.

Of course if you hate tailoring, then a tuxedo suit is not for you. If you look terrible in olive, then skip the utility jacket. If you live on an isolated farm, a little black dress probably isn't the best investment. <u>Look honestly at how you live</u>—and at your body shape—and shop accordingly. Don't buy anything that only works for best. <u>This is a seven-day-a-week wardrobe.</u> That little black dress should be as good for day as night. That tuxedo jacket is going to be worn with jeans for casual drinks with a girlfriend.

Relatedly, don't buy anything that is even slightly uncomfortable. You want clothes that enable you, not impede you. Anything you can't stride out in, or breathe deeply in, is not for you. That is not—thank goodness—what being a 21st-century woman is about. Again, it's that clear <u>head thing. Our clothes should leave us free to think about other matters; to live our lives to the fullest. Shop smart. Then enjoy.</u>

This doyenne's dozen is only a starting point, needless to say. Knowing myself as I do—the life I lead, what suits my shape, what makes me feel like me—I would add a floral dress, a patterned blouse, a jumpsuit, a shearling vest, a bright blazer, a couple more cashmere sweaters at the very least, some cropped pants in a neutral shade, a patterned floaty skirt, some embellished flats, and an array of earrings and lipsticks. I could get by on that very well indeed. Sure, it's a paragraph's worth of pieces, not a sentence, but I'd wager it's a fraction of what you currently have hanging in your closet. And in actuality, of course, it's a fraction of what I have, too.

Look honestly at how you live—and at your body shape—and shop accordingly.

51

I am not here to make you declutter to that degree. Though imagine the blissful liberation if one did. I know one magazine stylist who has swapped her candy shop of a closet for a rack of top-quality pantsuits. She says she feels emancipated. Whatever. I just know she looks great.

Nor am I here to tell you to utterly ignore trends. If you really love something that doesn't fit the classics brief, try it on in person and see if it suits you. Then give yourself a week of decompression time, try it on again, and if it still sparks joy, buy it. My only caution would be not to spend too much on anything that you suspect might prove transient.

On the other hand, invest as much as you can afford in the classics. And if, once you have worn a classic piece for a few weeks, you love it as much as you thought, and are worried it won't last indefinitely, buy several. (I am talking tees and sneakers at this point, not tuxedos.) But, to reiterate, don't splurge on trends unless you have money to burn, and who, quite frankly, has that?

"Fashion fades, only style remains the same," Coco Chanel once said. Find your own sense of style, and that fairy-tale ending is yours for the wearing.

NICE AND EASY DOES IT

Ease. That's what pulling together the oh-so elusive happy-ever-after wardrobe can deliver for you. Ease in the way you look. Ease in the way you feel. Just as importantly, it will make getting dressed in the morning simple, too, transforming it from a chore into a pleasure, and a swift one at that. Classic pieces such as a trench coat and a Breton top are likely to help you find your way to fashion freedom. But only if you love them. The happy-ever-after wardrobe is, at its name suggests, about what YOU love, which might be something else entirely.

There's nothing more versatile than a colorful jacket, which will change up weekday and weekend wear with equal aplomb.

Invest in the best-quality knitwear you can. Buy right and it will look as good on you today as five years down the line.

No for me

yes!

No white boots uh!

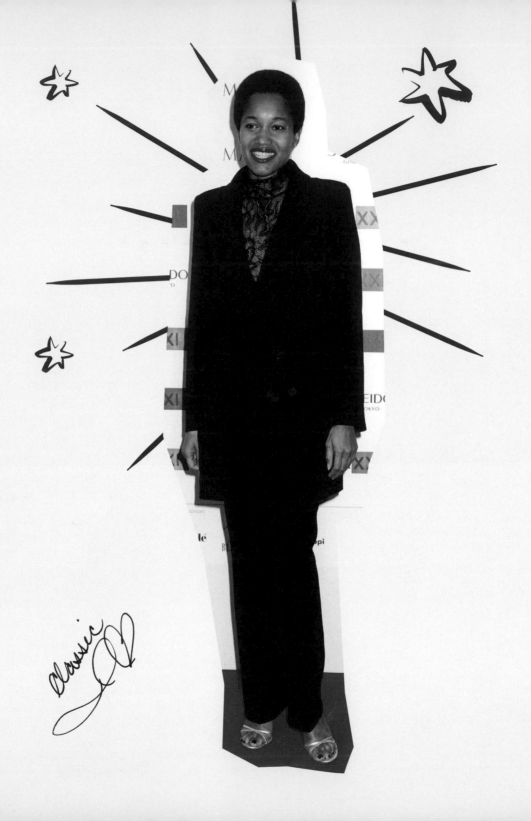

3

Boosting
the
Basics

BLACK AND BEYOND

It's all very well, the notion of Fashion with a capital F. But what we mainly need are basics, essentials, neutrals. Call them what you will, they are what we wear most of the time; they are our wardrobe nuts and bolts. They are the clothes that don't make demands of us, but answer the demands we make of them. They can be worn on different days, as part of different outfits.

That's why tracking down the perfect example of one of them—black pants, for example—is the consummate style success. But how to get the most out of these heavy-lifters without looking boring? That's always the risk when you buy plain, you buy basic, you buy—above all, black. How to boost those basics, elevate those essentials, nuclearize those neutrals?

THE B(L)ACK STORY

First up, black. It can prove the most loyal of fashion friends, but beware: overdo it and the ultimate non-color might just turn frenemy. Used judiciously it confers chic and—on a more practical level—oodles of bang for buck, in that it goes with everything in your wardrobe, and so not only scores high on that key price-per-wear scale, but also stretches the rest of what's in your closet further.

Yet wear too much of it, wear it head to toe in other words—with the marked exception of the little black dress—and it may just make you disappear. That, after all, was its historic purpose. Mourners wore it, a practice that dates back to the Roman Empire when the so-called *toga pulla* adopted by the recently bereaved was a dark gray or brown. Servants wore black, too. If a woman was living an unfettered existence, free of grief or the hard graft of a life in service, she never wore black.

When Coco Chanel sprang her little black dress on an unsuspecting world in 1926, it was nothing short of a revolution. Here was a servant's dress retooled to be fit for the lady of the manor. Indeed the designer exhorted her wealthy clients to "dress as plainly as their maids." Here was a bravura sleight of hand, which turned class codes on their head, which proved that less

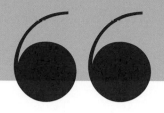

I imposed black; it is still going strong today, for black wipes out everything else around.

—COCO CHANEL

Less is more

really could be more. Or as Chanel put it, that "Elegance is refusal." (Her rival Paul Poiret saw things rather differently. "What has Chanel invented?" he asked at the time. "De luxe poverty.")

Only three decades earlier John Singer Sargent's famous portrait of "Madame X," actually a society belle called Madame Gautreau, had caused outrage not only for the sitter's come-hither *décolletage*, but also for her garb's blackness, which was considered indecent when worn by a woman not in mourning. Since then, due to the tragedy of World War I, mourning clothes had been worn on an unprecedented scale. So, though black was still—more than ever—linked with mourning, it was also less rare.

Vogue described that first little black dress as "Chanel's Ford," after Henry Ford's similarly revolutionary Model T car of the same era. Here was "the frock that all the world will wear," it prophesied. It was right. And nearly a century on, our love affair with the little black dress continues.

"I imposed black; it is still going strong today, for black wipes out everything else around," is how Chanel put it. But it's more complicated than the late designer suggests. She is both right and wrong. Play it right and black can "wipe out everything else." Get it wrong and it can wipe you out.

Black is a uniform. Which is both its strength and its weakness.

HI-VIS DRESSING

Does the Queen wear black? Nope. Do women in the public eye, be they politicians or movie stars? Not usually. They wear color— in the case of Her Majesty, often eye-poppingly bright color. Why? Because they want to stand out, not blend in. Theirs is a form of hi-vis dressing designed—like those fluorescent jackets worn by everyone from road workers to airport staff—to get them seen; to get them noticed.

As the Queen once memorably observed, "If I wore beige, nobody would know who I am." And what was the first fashion lesson learned by Samantha Cameron, the wife of the former British Prime Minister David Cameron, when she found herself in the public eye? "I couldn't wear black when I was with him because it looked as if we were going to a funeral," laughs the self-confessed neutrals lover. (Another problem, more specific to her: "I kept merging into the Number 10 door.")

Of course, when it comes to the film industry, there was a change of gear during the early months of #MeToo and #TimesUp, from late 2017 onward. At first the all-black dress code on the red carpet was inspired, a way for women to express their solidarity with others who had spoken out about abuse, and to signal the seriousness of a situation that had to change. This was a matter of life and death: what better color to signal that than black? Indeed, worn en masse at events like the Golden Globes, the LBD became a kind of hi-vis dressing all its own.

But then it risked turning into something else. Indeed, the original instigators had never planned for it to stick around. The #TimesUp "initiative was launched on the red carpet but was never intended to live there," said the TV writer and producer Shonda Rimes, best known for *Grey's Anatomy*.

As the designer Donatella Versace observed to me recently— while clad head-to-toe in body-con baby-blue—"I am very happy that #MeToo happened, but I didn't agree about everyone dressing in black." Why not? "Because that means you are changing yourself," she continued. "#MeToo is not about that. It is about saying, 'This is Me.'"

Again, take note. Chanel said she "imposed black." Black can indeed present like an imposition; like an erasure of individuality. Black is a uniform. Which is both its strength and its weakness.

There is also the question of how black works with your complexion. Your skin undertone may be cool, warm, or neutral, and in the next chapter you will find out how to determine which is which (see p.79). Black works well with cool complexions, and most neutral complexions, while a warm complexion would often be better off with a different, softer dark shade.

A Little navy dress boy yay!!

HOW TO LIFT YOUR LBD

Don't panic, though. I am not going to tell you to swear off black, not even when worn head to toe. As I said, I will allow you a little black dress, or two; even three. Indeed, buy well and the so-called LBD is the ultimate ever-after piece. What greater proof of its superlativeness than that it has its very own acronym? Though I would argue that—complexion-pending, as discussed—an LND, a little navy dress, can get you just as far.

I have an LBD in my wardrobe that dates from the 1970s, another from the 1990s, and they both look just as *au courant* as the one I bought last year. But take note of how Coco Chanel wore her most famous creation: with half a dozen strands of pearls. No danger of fading to gray, or rather black, with accessories like that.

Always animate your beloved LBD similarly, by way of look-at-me jewelry and/or shoes and/or bag and/or makeup, be it a statement lip or smoky eye. (Never overdo it with both. Plus, again, go for glam makeup and relaxed hair, or relaxed makeup and glam hair, not both.)

What's great about the LBD is that it offers a kind of blank canvas, which you can then ornament as you see fit. You don't have to stress about the dress, and can have fun with the add-ons. It may also, conversely, offer a way to have fun with the frock itself, because black's inherent classiness has the ability to render a fashion-forward number more user-friendly. An LBD can encompass lace, mesh, sparkle, frills, and still—if you pick it right—look chic. My most recent addition is an on-trend fantasia of filigree flounciness. In any other hue it would be too much; so fashionable as to be out of fashion five minutes later. In black it looks almost classic, and I am confident I will get a decade's wear out of it at least.

An LBD can encompass lace, mesh, sparkle, frills, and still—if you pick it right—look chic.

Stealth stupendousness, that's what the best kind of LBD can deliver. But you can make it more spectacular still with one or two eye-catching add-ons.

LITTLE BLACK DRESS

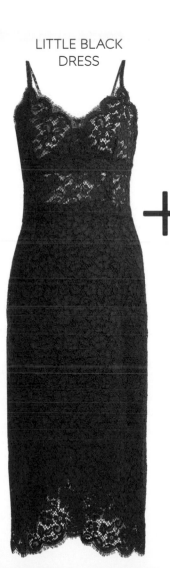

LOOK-AT-ME JEWELRY

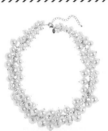

OR

STATEMENT LIP

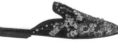

OR

KILLER SHOES

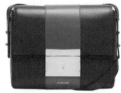

OR

GORGEOUS BAG

The BTS

A black tuxedo suit is another classic. Don't take it from me. Take it from devotees as diverse as Carey Mulligan, Halle Berry, Lauren Hutton, and—its original gender-bending advocate—the late Marlene Dietrich. Why the BTS hasn't become another acronym the well-dressed woman holds close to her heart is beyond me. Perhaps because it might be too easily confused with a BLT, or worse.

But, again, the tuxedo suit needs a lift: a silken blouse in white or cream, or a jewel shade; perhaps some splashy jewelry, and/or a silk scarf worn under the collar; something fantastic in the footwear department, though just what exactly that might be is entirely your call.

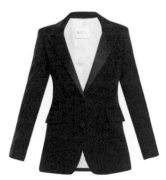
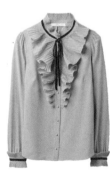
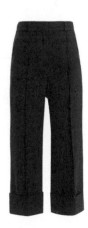

IT'S ALL IN THE DETAIL

If I am not wearing either an LBD or BTS (see left), I limit myself to one black item per outfit. If I wear a black jacket—perhaps that tuxedo jacket again—I wear a contrasting bottom half; perhaps jeans, perhaps a bright pleated skirt, perhaps brocade pants. If I wear black pants or a black skirt, I have fun with my top half, perhaps with an embroidery-strewn sweater, an embellished jacket, or a patterned blouse. The black bit is the bit you don't have to worry about: this—as with the LBD—is its secret power. As Samantha Cameron says, "put on a pair of black trousers with a heel and you suddenly feel put together; it gives you instant confidence." Then you use that confidence to turn things up with the rest of your look: to boost that basic; to "nifty-fy" (technical term) that neutral.

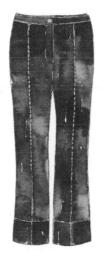

> "

What I am always on the look out for are essentials that have been upgraded in some way.

What I am always on the look out for are essentials that have been upgraded in some way. Like black pants with white stitching and buttons, or a hem which has been tweaked, maybe cropped, with a decorative trim or side buttoning, maybe ankle-length, with a slit or stepped cuff. Like a black skirt with statement pockets, or an interesting fabric texture, or an intricate waistline or hemline.

Or how about pants with military side-striping? In the last couple of years these have proved themselves to be a prime example of a permatrend. Permatrends are always good to embrace, because they make you appear current, but—due to the fact that they aren't going anywhere fast—don't risk you seeming out of date five minutes later (see Chapter 1).

Boosted Basics

All of these are boosted basics. And boosted basics are the key to a wardrobe that looks good but also works hard. They are basics because they are simple, wearable pieces that go with everything, everyday, everywhere. They are boosted because there is something special about them; a point of difference that makes them more than just another black skirt or pair of pants.

Go for the same approach with your top half, searching out interest-endowing detail. A contrasting collar on a shirt or jacket, an embellishment, or a textured fabric. Be we talking top half or bottom, special fabrics work wonders. Velvet, brocade, satin. Perhaps a juxtapositioning of two, or even three on one garment. Perhaps a detailing on an otherwise plain wool crepe.

I have a wool jacket that is subtly embossed with a snakeskin texture. It's so stealth that you might not immediately notice it, but it turns that jacket from nothing-much to knock-out. Yet it's a jacket that still goes with everything, so that I can—and frequently do—wear it with my more in-your-face separates. Like my silver brocade trousers, by way of one particularly noteworthy example. (What can I say? I am in fashion.) While I am not sure how I will feel about those trousers when I hit my 80s, I know I'll still be wearing that jacket.

Or you can stick with a plain black top half, and add the prerequisite stardust by way of jewelry or a bright lipstick or scarf. A black crew neck or silk tee and some chunky school-of-Coco faux pearls would be enough to outclass pretty much any opposition you might care to imagine.

FROM CROW TO PEACOCK

If you are really deft with this kind of mixing and matching within all-black parameters, you might even be able to pull off a separates-based head-to-toe look. Because the good news is that in the 21st century, fashion rules—including my own—are made to be broken. But, to reiterate: proceed with caution. The front row at Fashion Weeks around the globe used to be full of all-black wearers. The fashion critic Suzy Menkes observed how in the

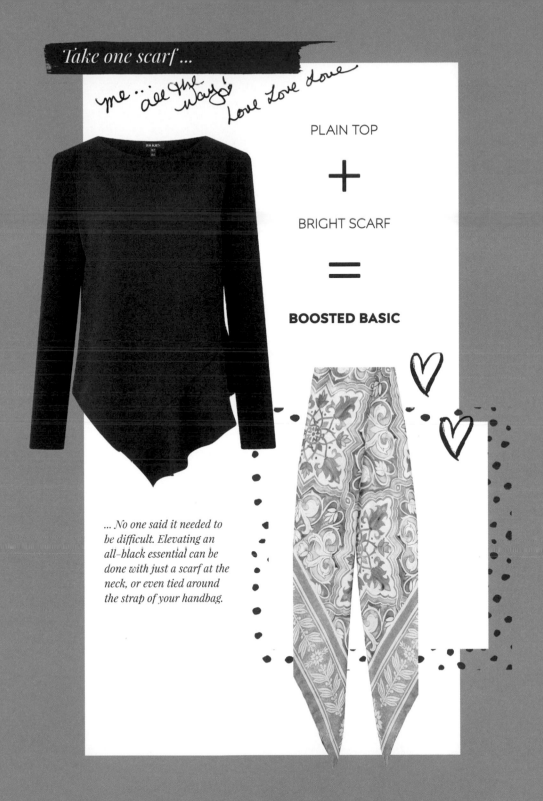

me ... all the way!
Love Love Love

PLAIN TOP

+

BRIGHT SCARF

=

BOOSTED BASIC

... No one said it needed to be difficult. Elevating an all-black essential can be done with just a scarf at the neck, or even tied around the strap of your handbag.

LBD check-up

Take a long, harsh look at your dress every so often and make sure it is still serving you well. Ask yourself a few simple questions:

♡ *Is it still working for me?*
♡ *Does it still fit?*
♡ *Does it need the hem slightly shortened or let out?*
♡ *Is it still black, or has it gone "off"?*

Black is a color that can age badly, turning an unsavory shade that might be blaown (brown-ish), blellow (yellow-ish), or blay (gray-ish). Not a good look.

Tweak or chuck—yes, chuck—accordingly.

1990s the fashion pack was described as looking like "black crows … 'Whose funeral is it?' passers-by would whisper with a mix of hushed caring and ghoulish inquiry."

In other words, even the experts get black wrong. Who wants to channel crow chic? Not me. That's partly why it's all changed among the fashion pack. Though it's also to do with the rise of Instagram, which has made some of the women who gather to watch the models as photographed as the models themselves. Now, says Menkes, "the people outside shows are more like peacocks than crows." The crows have figured out that some more exotic plumage might serve them better, in other words. Some front-row folk still wear black, sure, but they leaven it with color, even if that color is only in the form of another, less austere neutral.

KNOWING YOUR NEUTRALS

Other neutrals can actually be easier. Navy, olive, camel, brown, and gray, plus the neutral wild card you won't have been expecting, eggplant purple—these are your dark sextet. The ones that work best for you will be determined by whether your skin undertone is cool, warm, or neutral (see p.79), though there is likely to be an iteration of almost every shade—cooler, or more blue; warmer or more yellow/orange—that will make it suit you. Cream and white are your shining lights—the former if you are warm or neutral, the latter cool—though a true pure white will work on almost everyone.

All eight are wardrobe-workhorses in waiting. And they may well serve you better than black, which can be the least flattering of the bunch when worn directly next to the skin, especially as you age and lose your natural pigment. Navy, olive, and cream in particular can be much kinder on the complexion, and offer just the same versatility when it comes to mixing and matching with the rest of your wardrobe. No surprise that these three have become favorites with the fashion crowd.

What's more, worn head to toe they don't risk turning into that same cloak of invisibility as does black. Though, of course, white and cream have other risks of a stain-related nature. Also be aware

cream – warm + neutral skin tone

white for cool skin tone

that they, like black, have dozens of iterations, so make sure your theoretically matching separates complement each other rather than endow a low-grade seasickness. Thankfully these are shades that tend to distort far less over time than black.

Bear in mind, too, that they can be mixed up with brights with almost as much versatility as black can. Red, yellow, pink, lilac: just four of the summer-day hues that work well with navy and olive. Practically everything works with white and cream. Camel, brown, and gray can risk appearing wallflower, but not if you lift, lift, lift with crisp white at the very least or, better still, a splash or two of color. Brown and pale blue? Lovely. Camel and crisp green? ✓ Delicious. Gray with purple? Yes please. ✓

Or try mixing neutrals. Olive and black. Camel and navy. White or cream with black or navy is the ultimate classic combo of course, and there are some similarly timeless prints—be it polka dots or Prince of Wales check—which add interest while still ticking the "classic" box. If you want to push things a bit further though, how about polka dot plus check? A spotted blouse under a chessboard jacket perhaps. Or differently scaled iterations of the same pattern; a fine check skirt paired with a more amped-up check jacket, say? Both pieces might be mono, or one might

Very French - Navy & Black Combo ✓

❝

Try the once-verboten combination of navy and black, which is now proving itself to be another permatrend among the denizens of the front row.

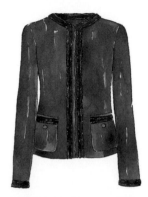

introduce some color. Either way: very chic, very now. I often wear a green and white houndstooth scarf layered under a monochrome jacket in the same pattern. Subtle, but it always gets me compliments. (See Chapter 7 for more ideas on mixing-and-non-matching.)

Ready to push things further still? Don't dismiss the once-verboten combination of navy and black, which is now proving itself to be another permatrend among the denizens of the front row. Contrast neutrals can work brilliantly, and there's much less room for error than clash-matching brights and/or patterns (see Chapter 4). I have an olive jacket—another front-row go-to—which does the hard work, such as it is, for me, by way of black appliqué at each shoulder. I have another, a tweedy affair, that is navy with a black trim. Genre-busting color-juxtapositioning delivered for me the second I put it on my shoulders.

It's addictive stuff. That's probably why I have just bought a pair of olive chinos pimped with black spots. I will be wearing them with my black tuxedo jacket.

Basics definitively boosted, thank you very much.

mix neutrals: Olive/Black
Camel/Navy   white/cream w Black/
                              Navy

Polka Dots
Prince of Wales check } are classic neutrals.

Polka Dot + a check?
Different scale of prints together

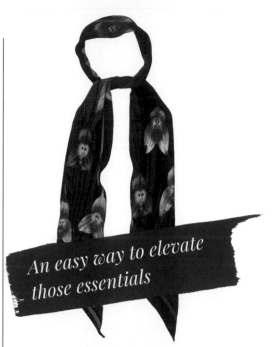

An easy way to elevate those essentials

72

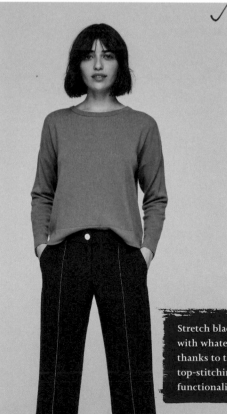

Navy plus navy plus navy. Could run the risk of looking like a school uniform, but not when one of those navies is patterned, and another is amped up with a pretty brooch.

Stretch black pants you can wear with whatever you choose— but thanks to the contrast button and top-stitching—don't look like a functionality-fueled compromise.

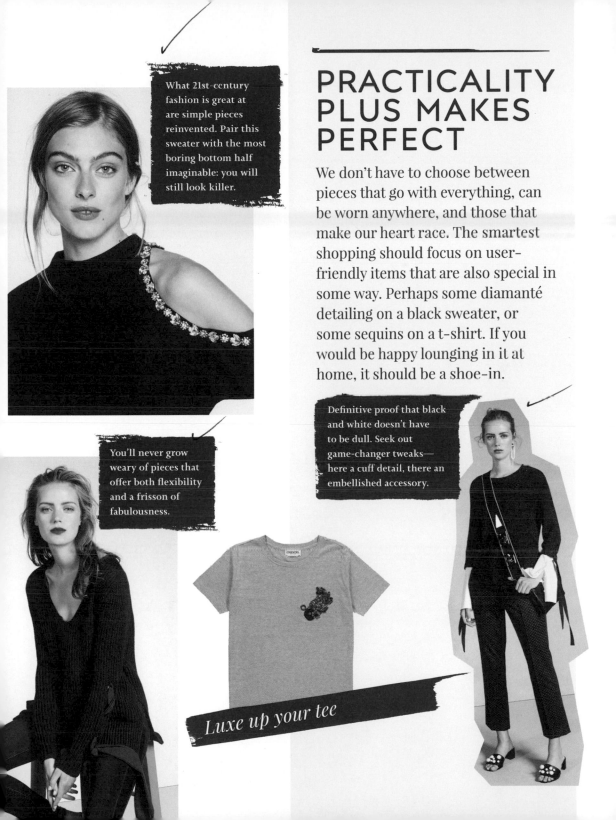

What 21st-century fashion is great at are simple pieces reinvented. Pair this sweater with the most boring bottom half imaginable: you will still look killer.

PRACTICALITY PLUS MAKES PERFECT

We don't have to choose between pieces that go with everything, can be worn anywhere, and those that make our heart race. The smartest shopping should focus on user-friendly items that are also special in some way. Perhaps some diamanté detailing on a black sweater, or some sequins on a t-shirt. If you would be happy lounging in it at home, it should be a shoe-in.

Definitive proof that black and white doesn't have to be dull. Seek out game-changer tweaks— here a cuff detail, there an embellished accessory.

You'll never grow weary of pieces that offer both flexibility and a frisson of fabulousness.

Luxe up your tee

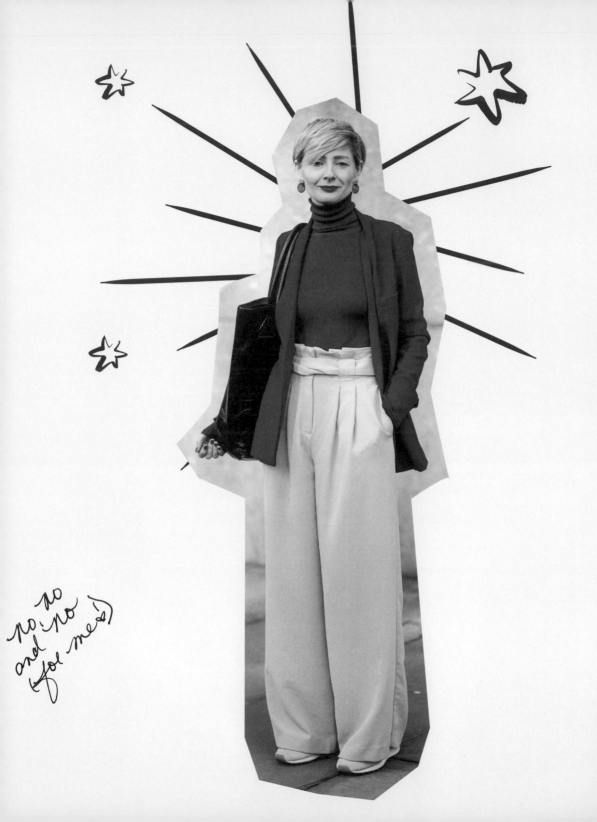

no no
and no
(for me)

4

Color Me
Beautiful,
Pattern Me
Perfect

HOW TO GO
OVER THE RAINBOW

How much do you have in your wardrobe? Color and pattern, that is. Some of us embrace it, but more of us eschew it. Why? Because we fear that we will get it wrong and end up in something that doesn't suit us. The thing is, you can pick wrong when it comes to plain neutrals, too. Indeed, color and pattern can actually prove far simpler to nail when dressing to flatter your silhouette. What's more, they are two of the easiest ways to change up your appearance. They can transform the way you look and feel. They can change the vibration of a room when you walk into it, and continue to resonate long afterward, when that room and what happened in it are just a memory.

Let me share with you a couple of examples of the power of color. What do you think of when you read the words *Atonement* green? Something very precise, I imagine. That wonderful emerald hue worn by Keira Knightley in the film of Ian McEwan's novel. I was talking at a fashion event recently and someone in the audience asked me for advice about what shoes she should wear with the "*Atonement* green wedding dress" she had picked out. There were over a hundred women in the room and we all knew immediately what she meant, and audibly swooned with delight. Would we have done the same should she have referred to a white dress, or black, or navy? Of course not!

Then there is one of my favorite books, Rosamond Lehmann's *Invitation to the Waltz*. It's a coming of age tale, the story of Olivia Curtis' first dance, told through a coming of color, the story of the "flame-colored silk" dress she will wear to it, chosen by her elder sister, to her mother's consternation. Things happen when Olivia wears that dress. Things tend to when you dress brightly.

"The patches of color splashing one's wardrobe's history were as rare … as roses in December," the 17-year-old Olivia muses. "Each one remained vivid in memory: isolated accidents, shocks of brightness: a crimson ribbon slotted through an early white party frock … an orange Liberty scarf on a straw hat; a curious coat of violet …." Her vow: "Now that I am grown up and can choose my own clothes, I'll wear bright colors always."

"

Now that I am grown up and can choose my own clothes, I'll wear bright colors always.

—OLIVIA, *INVITATION TO THE WALTZ*, ROSAMOND LEHMANN

Why not embellish our own lives similarly? Not least because color is the female superpower. Literally. Neuroscientists have determined that women have a larger color vocabulary than men: we are more adept at perceiving gradations of hue. Then there are the super-seers, so-called tetrachromats, who can distinguish a hundred million colors, each familiar shade fracturing a hundred times over. Several species of fish, bird, and mammal are tetrachromats, but so far only one human has been found. You guessed it, she's female, an unnamed doctor from the north of England.

But color is also our superpower because we get to wear it, to enjoy it, and to use it in a way that is not open to all but the most adventurous men. In a world which is more "stage-play" than ever, courtesy of social media, it's color that will make you pop, make you stand out. And standing out is not a bad thing, if you know that you're looking great. It can help you make friends and influence people, both in your working life and off-duty. It can help you develop—and enjoy—who you are. Color, the right color, can be an expression of self; more than that, a celebration of self. And the same goes for pattern, the right pattern.

SPECTRUM STYLE

How to find the right hue/s for you? Silhouettes are always going to be complicated because an inch up or down on a waistband, or in and out on a peplum, can change the perimeters of a particular ensemble far more than you might think. But once you've determined your skin tone (for colors) and your frame size (for patterns) you'll pretty much have nailed what works for you.

Skin tone first. It is this more than anything else that determines what colors you will look good in. Are you warm, cool, or neutral? To be precise, what we're actually talking about is skin undertone. Because someone fair-skinned can have warm undertones, as is the case with Claire Danes, and someone dark-skinned can be cool, to wit Lupita Nyong'o.

Confused? There are some simple tests to figure out what you are. If one or two don't lead to a definitive conclusion either way, keep going until you find the ones that do.

FIND YOUR SKIN UNDERTONE

First, hold a piece of pure white paper next to your unmade-up face and look in the mirror. How does your skin compare? If it looks pink, rosy, or blue you have a cool skin tone. If it appears more yellow, green, or light brown then you are probably warm. If your skin looks gray or ashen, then you are most likely neutral.

Standing out is not a bad thing if you know you're looking great. It can help you make friends and influence people.

Next, examine the veins on the inside of your arm. If they appear blue/purple you're probably cool; if they appear green, you are warm; if it's hard to decide you are probably neutral.

Usually if you have blue, green, or gray eyes with naturally blonde, brown, or black hair, all with undertones of silver, ash, blue, or violet, you are probably cool. If you have brown, amber, or hazel eyes with naturally strawberry blonde, red, brown, or black hair, all with undertones of gold, red, orange, or yellow, you are likely to be warm.

What else? Cool tones tend not to tan easily, warm tones do; neutral could go either way. Cool suits silver jewelry, warm gold, and neutral has the pick of the bling.

WHAT SHADES SUIT YOU?

When it comes to colors you'll be unsurprised to learn that cools look good in cool shades, warms in warm ones, and that neutrals have more latitude. So if you are cool seek out hues that make you think of winter and/or the sea: blues, blue-greens, purples,

I don't always agree with these comments →

magentas, and blue-based reds. When it comes to neutrals, favor black, bright white, navy, and cool grays.

Warm tones should pick yellows, oranges, browns, yellow-greens, orange-based reds, and softer neutrals such as creams, taupes, and gentle grays.

Some neutrals can go anywhere over the rainbow, subject to the usual full-length mirror test (see p.22). Others tend to look better in shades that don't overwhelm their tones, like a dusky pink rather than a magenta, a blue that's soft rather than electric, and neutrals that include off-whites, mid-range grays, coffee, and black. All neutrals will shine in an all-singing, all-dancing true red, i.e. one that has neither blue nor orange undertones.

There are also a handful of hues that work well for almost everyone. Pure white, for example, goes with all skin tones. If a particular item doesn't look good on you it will probably be because it has cool or warm undertones. A shade of teal that is the right balance of blue and green flatters everyone, and a light blush pink brings out a glow in all complexions. A great universal neutral is eggplant, which accentuates rather than overpowers, and which also adds interest.

Distressed to learn that a color you love isn't for you? There may be a version of it that will be, one that's tweaked to skew warm or cool. And if there isn't? Wear it as an accent, especially if it is not next to the skin, perhaps in the form of a belt or handbag.

> **A great universal neutral is eggplant, which accentuates rather than overpowers.**

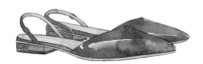

THE PRINT PRINCIPLE

Pattern next. Why does frame size matter? Because that's what tells you which scale of pattern is right for you. Measure your wrists way to make the user-friendly clothes we all demand in our busy lives look interesting, different. If you still can't get your head around the idea then classics like polka dots or checks are a good way in, again chosen according to your lines.

One approach that delivers a particularly contemporary feel is to wear traditionally winter prints such as animal print and houndstooth over summer fabrics like silk. Indeed, the boundaries between what's "winter" and what's "summer" are merging more and more, and there's no more modern look than to pair, say, animal-print pajama bottoms with a vast winter woolly sweater come Christmas Day.

A second singularly 21st-century route in is the clash-matching of pattern and/or scale. You can buy a single piece like a dress that delivers this for you, but always remember to consider both the relationship between the patterns and your frame size and shape, plus whether the arrangement of the contrast patterns draws attention to the right bits of your particular body. (A bright and/or big print will attract the eye to a greater degree than a more restrained one.)

If you're feeling brave, you can give the clash-matching a try by way of separates. Two fairly fail-safe routes in: Stick to one type of classic pattern in two different scales and/or colorways—two houndstooth checks; two polka dots—or mix two different patterns but in one chiming color—so a green and white striped shirt with green and white floral trousers, for example.

Whatever, however, you choose to embrace color and pattern, wear them with confidence. More than that, enjoy!

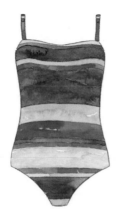

66 *no patterns for me – no, no and no.*

A swimsuit or bikini with horizontal stripes across the bust can work wonders for the less well-endowed.

these are just plain ugly

84

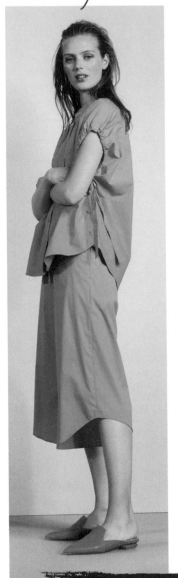

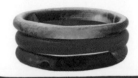

A stack of bangles is an easy-peasy add-on

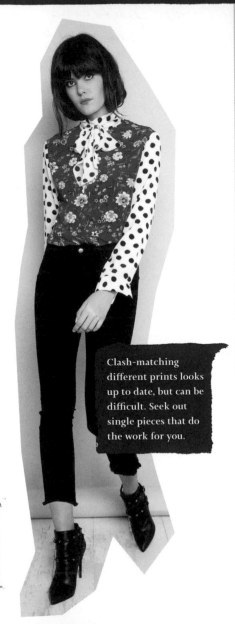

Clash-matching
different prints looks
up to date, but can be
difficult. Seek out
single pieces that do
the work for you.

Opposites really do attract.
Shades that face each other
on the color wheel—like
blue and orange—always
look good.

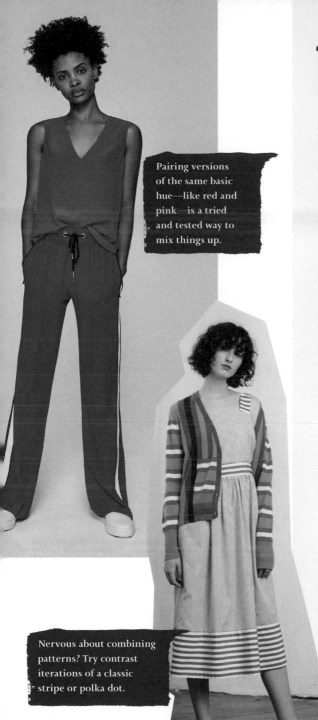

Pairing versions of the same basic hue—like red and pink—is a tried and tested way to mix things up.

Nervous about combining patterns? Try contrast iterations of a classic stripe or polka dot.

RAINBOW WARRIOR

Expanding your style toolkit so that you can dress confidently in different colors and patterns is going to make you look modern. It's also going to give you—and other people—so much pleasure. It can seem overwhelming at the beginning. But the guidelines in this chapter make it easy to find out your skin undertone, become friends with the color wheel, and learn a few pattern-mixing tricks. The world—and the spectrum—is your oyster!

One jewel-bright piece is all an outfit needs

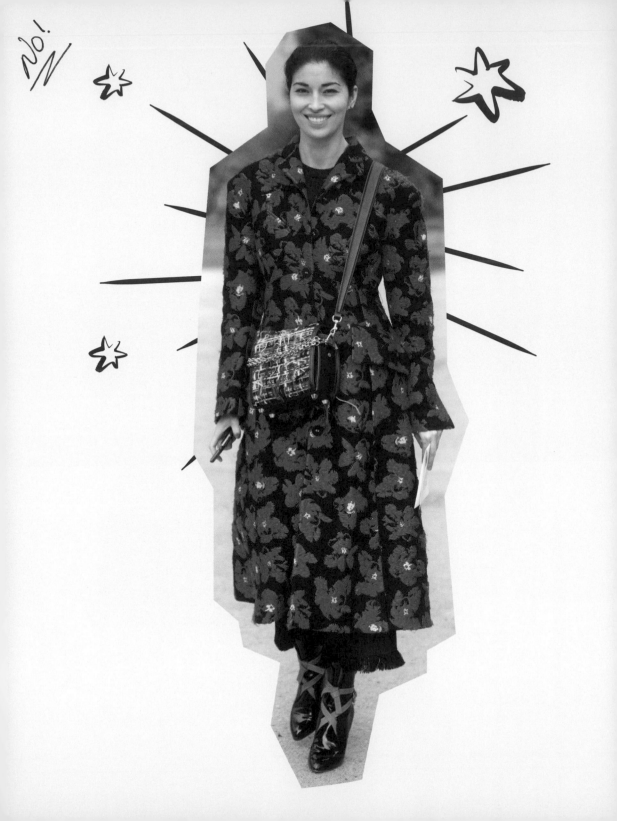

5

The Fit-Bag
and the
Statement
Coat

PRESENTING YOUR MOST
STYLISH SELF TO THE WORLD

The two easiest ways to tell the world at large something about yourself by way of what you have about your person is via your bag or, weather depending, your coat. That's why if there are two items it's worth making an effort with, it's these.

We live in the era of the it-bag. The handbag has become the most totemic fashion purchase most women make, and often the most expensive. Why? Because women are out in the world—and, more specifically, in the workplace—like never before. After centuries in which the majority of our time was spent at home, we are on the move. In the 1930s, the biggest-selling item of clothing at Marks & Spencer was an apron. Housework was what defined most women's lives. The handbag is indicative of an era when we females are literally, not to mention metaphorically, in transit.

And when we are on the move, we—in contrast to men—like to have a few accoutrements on hand, not least because relentless beauty marketing tells us that we should. How ironic then that—unlike men—our clothes tend not to be designed to carry anything. (Clothes without pockets are a *bête noire* of mine, but pockets do, thankfully, seem to be on the rise at last.)

No wonder we started buying bags like never before, and no wonder the fashion industry—especially the luxury end—cottoned on to the fact that this was a way for them to make money. This is all surprisingly recent history. The Fendi baguette bag of 1997 was arguably the first it-bag. There have been countless it-bags since then, and there are no doubt countless more to come. These days, accessories—along with beauty—have become the bread and butter at most luxury brands.

This is why those brands want us to keep on buying it-bags, rather than find our fit-bag, by which I mean the bag that fits our personal style, that fits the realities of our daily life, and that is designed with functionality in mind, as well as fashion.

The problem with the it-bag is indicated by its name. If something is "it," that means it's only a matter of time before it's not-it. And that's not all. In my job I have been lucky enough over the years to test-carry any number of it-bags, many of them

"

Something ugly can be made better. Just put a fabulous coat on top.

—MICHAEL KORS

Arm candy–colored

If you are spending serious money on a handbag, the temptation is of course always to play it safe. Indeed, when it comes to practicality, to quality, to durability, you should do just that. But when it comes to color, I would urge non-caution. Black, taupe, navy, brown. I understand the appeal. But a more look-at-me hue of handbag can add interest to every outfit, and, precisely because it doesn't "go" with anything, can oddly work with everything. I call it matchy-non-matchy. And, trust me, it can be a real game changer.

Leopard-print is unbeatable at this. It's also hard to better a red handbag. Still not sure? How about a dark shade that is almost as sensible as those neutrals but much more interesting? Forest green, perhaps, or deep purple?

But if there is a particular bright that you love, that makes your heart lift every time you see it, why not buy it in bag form? It will be a ray of sunshine to brighten your mood every morning, even if it isn't in fact yellow.

Isn't that what this stuff should be about? Arm candy: the clue is in the name. Sweets for grown-ups. So buy yourself a bag that will make you smile, while also proving to be the workhorse that every modern woman needs.

extremely expensive. Remarkably, the majority of them had a clasp that was difficult to use, or a shape that gaped, or some other element of basic design that was unsatisfactory. Then there's the heaviness factor. If you have a $1,300 back-breaker in your wardrobe, that is where it will stay. However beautiful a bag is, if the functionality isn't there you won't use it. I speak from experience. So forget about the it-bag and start thinking fit-bag: the functional, forever-after it-bag. I promise you it's out there, and together we can find it.

WHAT TO LOOK FOR

It's key to buy the best quality you can, because a fit-bag is going to be your fairy-tale ending, accessories-wise; your knight in shining leather. In this we should think like our mothers, if not our grandmothers, and invest. But don't assume that because something is expensive it is good quality or, even if it is good quality, that it will age well.

Some amazing leathers damage easily. Beware of anything very smooth (unless it's patent, which is surprisingly practical) or, conversely, very rough, because both will show the inevitable scratches. I am a fan of calfskin, which looks great and is durable. And don't think you have to spend a lot of money, although don't think you can get away with super-cheap either. There are some boutique handbag brands that are producing top-notch products at $260 to $525, prices that should make the luxury brands ashamed.

However beautiful a bag is, if the functionality isn't there you won't use it.

Another thing to consider is the style of bag. Hands-free is the most-user friendly option for our busy 21st-century lives. A tote may seem wonderful in theory, but for me the day-to-day default is a cross-body every time. On days when I need to carry more— and we all know there always are those days—I also carry a tote, into which I can even put my cross-body should I want to. Double-bagging. A neat solution to our multi-faceted lives.

Friends who have larger chests have lamented the cross-body's divide and conquer tendencies, in which case the approach for you should be either a shoulder bag or even a new-generation fanny pack. (Yes, really. There are some lovely grown-up leather iterations available these days.) Canniest of all is to buy a bag that can adapt from cross-body to shoulder as your day/outfit/mood dictates. Some brands even offer a cross-body that converts to a fanny pack.

HOW TO FIND IT

In terms of size, the fashion industry is always trumpeting something new. Small one season, large the next, positively minuscule the one after. Ignore. Put everything you normally carry on the kitchen table. Evaluate whether you need it all. I have dramatically downsized in the last year, ditching my wallet and my planner. Despite being something of a Luddite, I have to concede that the fact I can now pay almost everywhere by card and/or phone, and have a calendar on my phone, has considerably lightened my daily load.

Put that final edit of items into a plastic carrier bag. Plonk it into your current handbag. You are now ready to go fit-bag shopping. You need to take your time over this, and you need to shop in-store not online. Or, to be more precise, you need to not-shop in-store two, maybe three, times before you actually buy. Scope out online first, but then go into the shop, over and over.

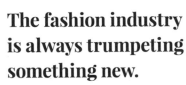

The fashion industry is always trumpeting something new. Ignore.

One key to being a successful shopper is to be an unembarrassable one. Make the clerk your friend. Have a laugh together about your retail geekery. Enjoy yourself. They will end up enjoying it, too. And you might find yourself with some useful information, like if said bag is going to be discounted someday soon.

A historical note

The first woman to become tired of carrying her bag in her hand was Coco Chanel back in the 1920s. It was this designer's persnicketiness—as well as creativity—that has made our lives so much easier in so many ways. Inspired by the straps on soldiers' bags, she added some to a bag she first launched in 1929, decades later reincarnated as the iconic 2.55.

Other celebrated it-bags take their names from their most famous devotee. The Hermès Kelly bag only became known as such two decades after its 1935 launch, when Grace Kelly used it to shield her pregnancy from reporters. The same brand's Birkin reputedly came about when the actress Jane Birkin was seated next to an Hermès executive on a plane in the mid-1980s, and observed that she needed a generous carryall.

Some took their name from something else entirely, most notably Fendi's baguette bag of 1997, which ended up selling like hotcakes rather than mere bread. One hundred thousand were bought in the first year.

Take out your plastic bag of must-have-withs and put it in the handbag you are eyeing up. No easier way to work out if it is the right size for you. Open and shut that clasp over and again and be brutally honest with yourself about whether the way it works really works for you. Put that bag on and hang out in the store with it, walking around, sitting down, taking it off, putting it back on. Again, is it ticking the boxes for you; really ticking the boxes?

Every time you go back to the store, wear something different than last time. Although there is ever more cohesion for many of us between our on-duty and off-duty wardrobes, there are still differences, and some of us in the more male-dominated professions continue to dress in a highly demarcated way. Make sure this bag does the job for you across the board. Of course, you could buy two different bags. But how much better to buy one? Or at the very least to buy two that work together, in best double-bagging style.

94

THE STATEMENT COAT

There's something else that's come along more recently that can—depending on your climate—work just as hard for you, and bring just as much joy. The statement coat. On the fall/winter catwalks of today—and even on the spring/summer ones—the savviest, most commercial designers present myriad outerwear options. Whereas once upon a time one coat per collection was enough, now half a dozen or more is par for the course.

What's changed? I spoke to designer Michael Kors, a past master season after season of high-end iterations of what I call coat candy. "Something ugly can be made better. Just put a fabulous coat on top," he told me. He's right. Despite the casualization of the world—or indeed because of it—most of us are game for a one-stop way to transform our yoga gear, or worse, into something that looks appropriate for a meeting on the run.

Sling a fabulous coat over your shoulders and it delivers like nothing else. That's why the wardrobes of many fashion women have a new emphasis on outerwear. They have cut back on everything else, but they have a collection of coats rather than just one or two.

keen look in New York

Don't want to wear a coat indoors at your local café, or wherever? Take that shoulder-slinging directive literally, wearing it over your shoulders without putting your arms through the sleeves. The fashion pack is all about this so-called "shoulder-robing." Sounds ridiculous at first, and it certainly takes a bit of getting used to, but once you've got the hang of it, I hereby pledge that shoulder-robing will add statement coat pizzazz without making you get hot under the collar.

What makes a coat a statement? It could be a color or pattern. A bright check, or that leopard print again. (What do you mean, I am obsessed?) The matchy-non-matchy principle is in play here once more. Pick well, and a coat that doesn't match anything will work mysteriously well across your entire wardrobe.

Still not convinced? Go for a more subtle approach. It might be distinctive buttons or a styling quirk. Or—a favorite of mine—a detachable collar that turns a plain black coat suddenly opinionated. Whatever you go for, make sure your statement coat, like your fit-bag, sparks joy.

Coat candy. Arm candy. They turn back the clock in the best possible sense, making you not only look younger but also feel younger. That's why these are two of the most life-enhancing fashion purchases you can make.

> ❝
> _____
>
> ## Shoulder-robing will add statement-coat pizzazz without making you get hot under the collar.

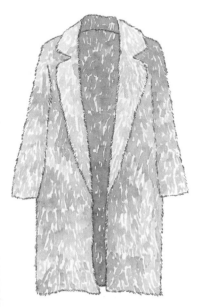

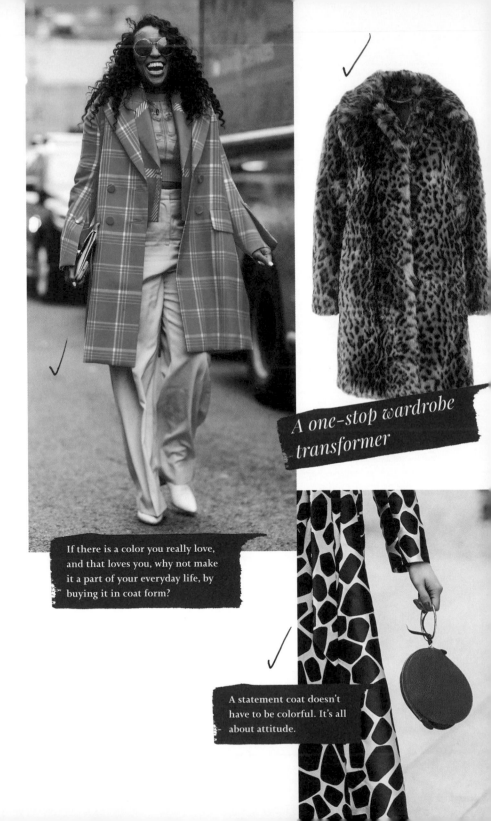

A one-stop wardrobe transformer

If there is a color you really love, and that loves you, why not make it a part of your everyday life, by buying it in coat form?

A statement coat doesn't have to be colorful. It's all about attitude.

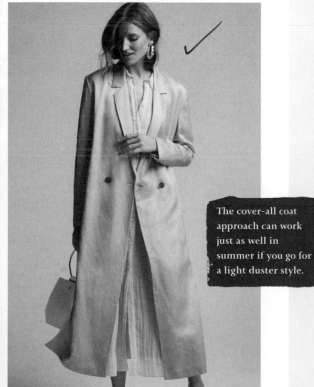

The fanny pack has come of age: not just grown up but chic, and super-practical if you don't need to carry much.

YOUR TWO FIRMEST FASHION FRIENDS

No items are going to work harder for you than your coat and your bag. They are going to make you look and feel great even if you are merely popping out to the corner store. They are going to disguise whatever is—or isn't—going on underneath. Because, sometimes, as we all know, life is just too short to change out of your gym gear, not to mention—on occasion—your pajamas. (Shhhh! Our little secret!) Look for color and pattern. That's what is going to turn a coat into a statement, a bag into a smile. But also focus on function, function, function. These are pieces that may look playful but, as I said, they need to graft as much as you do.

The cover-all coat approach can work just as well in summer if you go for a light duster style.

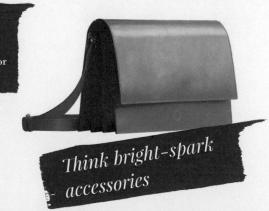

Think bright-spark accessories

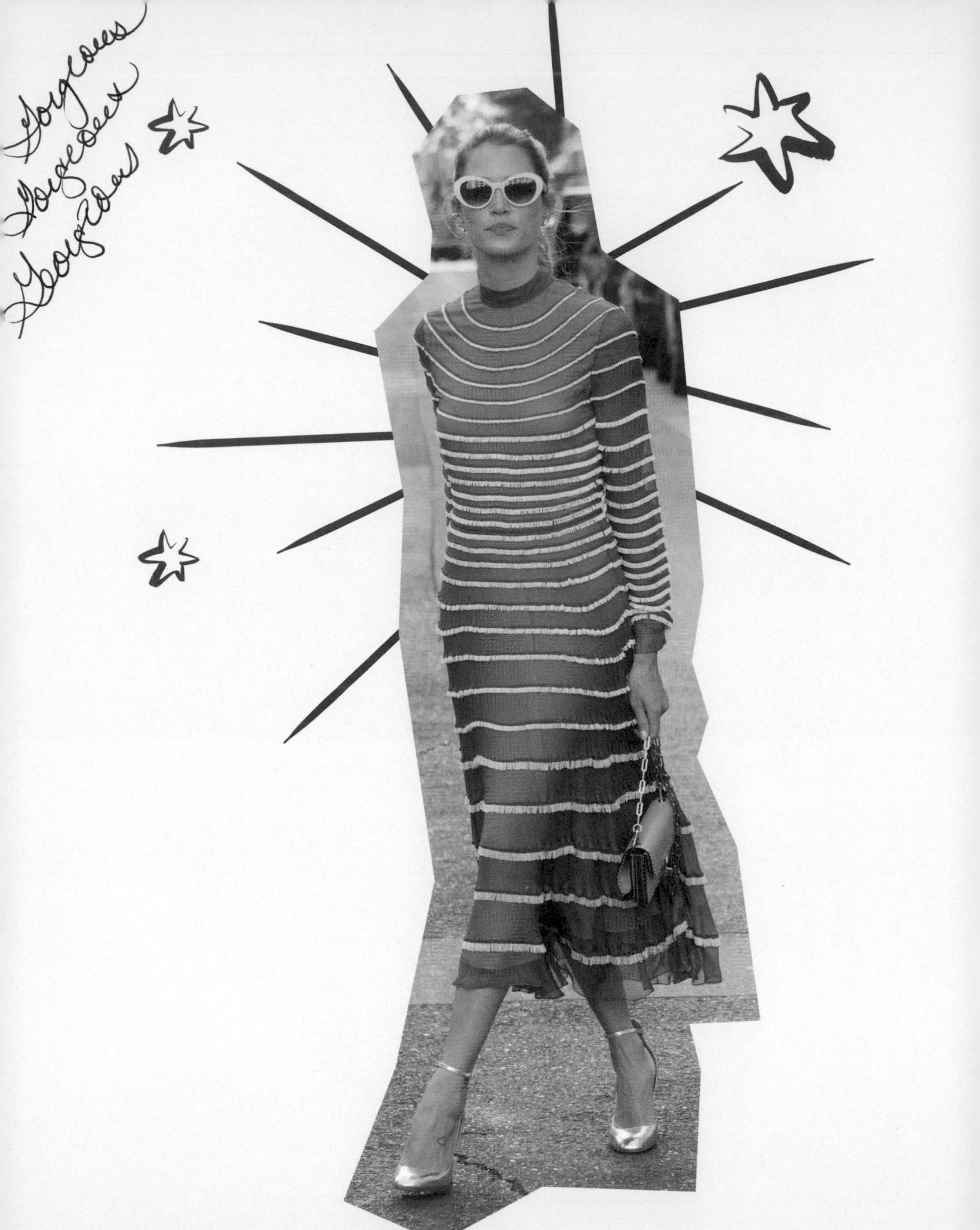
Gorgeous
Gorgeous
Gorgeous

6

Super-Heroine
Style

THE ONE-STOP LOOK, FROM
DRESSES TO JUMPSUITS

Throw on a dress, and you are immediately transformed. It is the wardrobe equivalent of Wonder Woman's garb-changing warp-spin, and it, too, can endow you with super-heroine powers, powers that may not help you slay baddies in the literal sense, but that can facilitate a more metaphorical variety of swathe-cutting, be it in the workplace or socially.

If you buy a dress that is right, the job is done, once and for all. You put it on. You look good. As the designer Carolina Herrera said to me a while back, clad in the perfect chambray shirtdress by way of illustration, "What does every woman look good in, whatever her age, whatever her size? A dress."

Diane von Furstenberg, who created her celebrated wrap dress in 1974, once observed to me, "I quickly realized I was selling confidence. It was an attitude. At a time of liberation." A dress, strange as it may seem, can set you free.

When a preternaturally stylish American friend of mine moved to London two decades ago she expressed bafflement. "Why do you Brits never wear dresses?" she asked. "Dresses are so much more simple than separates. They do all the work for you." Now many of us have embraced dresses once again. We just need to make sure to pick modern, and to wear modern.

Certainly separates are easier to get wrong. Pants that work well with one top can be unflattering with another. And don't get me started on skirts. A minefield. Plus, even a successful separates-based ensemble can seem try-hard if there are too many different elements.

On the other hand if you buy a dress that suits your body shape, it's hard to mess it up. So why do so many of us shy away from the ultimate in solution dressing? Why do some of us still consider a dress to be a special-occasion thing, rather than an every-day thing?

Maybe because there was a time when a dress was either formal or frumpy. On the one hand there was Holly Golightly's in *Breakfast at Tiffany's*: black, sleek, chic, but probably not that conducive to running for the bus. On the other there were Miss

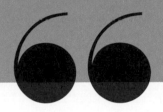

What does every woman look good in, whatever her age, whatever her size? A dress.

— CAROLINA HERRERA

Marple's: floral, a tad dowdy, and great for striding around sleuthing, but about as alluring as a tent. But now we have reached peak dress, in the sense that there is so much fabulosity out there to choose from.

You can make like Holly Golightly but still catch the number 23 bus courtesy of new-generation fabrics that offer imperceptible stretch. If you shop really well, you can even throw it in the washing machine afterward. (I always look for machine-washable—as well as pockets. But I have also found that a cool hand-wash will work for many items labeled dry-clean-only. It's become an annoying habit of fashion brands to cover their backs by declaring something dry clean only, when it actually isn't.)

Or you can embrace the new-gen floral, which has many features that Miss Marple would recognize but has been reinvented to be cool-girl. It was Demna Gvasalia, head honcho at the cult label Vetements, and recently also at the illustrious house of Balenciaga, who started it all back in 2015. "Everyone knew the vintage floral dress," he told me. "We looked at how to reinterpret it, how to make it look different, so that people would come to us to buy one instead." He kept the long sleeves and the mid-calf-length skirt, but he used strong, modern-looking prints, and added into the mix asymmetric hemlines and the occasional clash-match insert of a different fabric entirely.

That long-heard lament "Where are the dresses with sleeves?!" is no longer relevant, because they are everywhere.

Vetements dresses may not be for the faint-hearted, but there are more subtle iterations all over that will flatter whatever your age and size. That long-heard lament "Where are the dresses with sleeves?!" is no longer relevant, because they are everywhere. If you are slim you will look great in a loose, unwaisted take, but the rest of us might want to think about belting it.

THE A,B,C OF DRESSES

Some dress-related thoughts: That everyone looks good in a button-down style, and that if it's unwaisted and in a soft fabric it can do double-duty open and layered on top of jeans or plain trousers and a tee. A kimono dress—currently having something of a moment—offers this same versatility.

That a skirt-length that emphasizes one of the slimmest parts of your figure—namely your lower calves and ankles—is often the most flattering. Don't take it from me, take it from stylist Rebecca Corbin-Murray, who says this is one of her most important criteria when picking red carpet dresses for her clients. "The narrowest part of your leg is between your ankle and your mid-calf. If you have a dress that cuts you off there, and that also pulls you in at the waist, it is slimming and elongating."

Corbin-Murray and I shared disbelieving notes when we last met as to why, until very recently, so many of the more affordable brands insisted on offering dresses that were cut just above or below the knee, both cumbersome lengths for all but the most willowy of leg. Was it a money-saving initiative or sheer ignorance? We couldn't decide.

Certainly if you are prepared to spend money—lots of money, as Corbin-Murray's clients do—it becomes much easier. But, at a lower price point, things have finally changed. It is still all too easy to buy a dress that's an unflattering length, which must be why so many women continue to get this part of the equation wrong. A friend of mine who organizes weddings says the most common mistake she sees is for a woman to wear a dress that cuts her legs at the wrong place. But now, with all the affordable options we suddenly have to choose from, there are no excuses any more. Remember the towel test (see p.34). Find your happy place, skirt-length-wise.

WHY CROOKED CAN BE WONDERFUL

Not only is the so-called Vetements effect making it easier than ever to find longer skirts, the rise—and fall, and rise again—of the asymmetric hemline is also something to factor in. I didn't like the idea at all initially. As someone who endured a singularly crooked-hemmed childhood, courtesy of clothes that were bought with "room for growth" and then let down with—how shall I put this so as not to offend my mother?—a certain idiosyncrasy, why would I pay good money for similar?

Because an asymmetric hem adds a contemporary feel. You don't want anything too extreme or complicated, but a bit of a swoop and a dip ensures that—however flowery of fabric, long of sleeve, and chaste of neckline your dress is—there's not a whisper of old lady about your person.

As Justin Thornton, one half of the upscale British label Preen—purveyor of asymmetric perfection season after season—says, "It gives a dress an edge, and stops it looking too retro." And as Thea Bregazzi—his partner in design and in life—adds, "On a longer style it can be more flattering and less shortening than a straight hem." In other words, this is a way of having your cake and eating it. So don't dismiss it out of hand. A less edgy way to flash just enough flesh is courtesy of a slit or two.

The unified lines of a dress flatter like nothing else. But if you are a larger size, don't use a dress to swamp your form, as it will just end up making you look bigger. Instead rely on that ankle- and lower-calf-flashing. A straight-up-and-down shift dress tends not to do any favors to all but the super-skinny. Far better to have a dress with some shape, be it empire line or waisted. If you are big-busted you should also avoid the shelf effect by picking a style that has a *décolletage*, though not too much of one. It's you in your gorgeous entirety that you want to get looked at, not your cleavage alone.

A bit of a swoop and a dip ensures that there's not a whisper of old lady about your person.

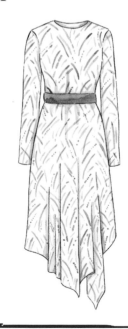

IF YOU'VE GOT IT, FLAUNT IT

If your upper arms are toned, you can make like Michelle Obama and flash that ultimate 21st-century female status symbol with a sleeveless style. Yet don't dismiss a sleeveless style out of hand if you aren't in love with your arms but are in love with everything else about that dress. Because although the appeal of the dress is those one-stop abilities, you can tweak it, too, with layers. The most straightforward approach is, of course, to wear a top layer, perhaps a lovely cardigan, or a luxe bomber. But you can also layer under a thin long-sleeved tee if the dress is in a suitably relaxed style, or Spanx's Arm Tights if it's more formal.

One more thing. Don't forget the power of footwear to reinvent a dress. The same dress worn with spindly lady-shoes or sneakers will present entirely differently. To generalize, the most modern approach is to wear a mid-heel that is on the chunky side for dressy—or perhaps an ankle boot or a platform sandal—and sneakers for casual. Flats or kitten heels could work for both.

DON'T DISMISS THE JUMPSUIT

There's another item of clothing that instantaneously transforms you, and that's the jumpsuit. Think about it. What is a jumpsuit but a dress with legs? It does all the hard work for you in exactly the same way, smoothing your lines, and making you look effortlessly pulled together. But it delivers something else, too—namely an injection of cool. A jumpsuit may once have been a utility workaday item worn by fighter pilots and mechanics, but in recent years it has been reinvented in upscale fabrics and sleek cuts.

Lots of women don't like the idea of a jumpsuit. But growing numbers—myself included—have become slightly obsessed. I have a 20-something friend who wears little else, from hipster denim to patterned silk, and a 60-something friend who favors tailored iterations in black and navy crepes. I have versions of all of these styles in my wardrobe, that's how much I love a jumpsuit, and they are some of my most complimented pieces. I layer a tee underneath, or even a super-thin sweater for extra warmth.

105

DRESS

+

SNEAKERS

=

CASUAL CHIC

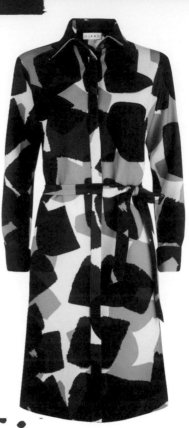

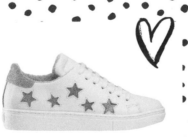

It's akin to an elixir of youth, having a pair of crisp white sneakers in your wardrobe. Wear them with an otherwise dressy ensemble and they can knock decades off your look.

What can I say? Things happen when you wear an LBJ.

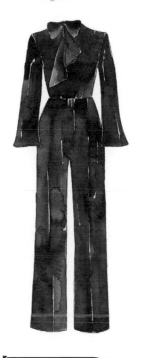

My favorite is probably my LBJ, my little black jumpsuit, of which I am sure Holly Golightly herself would have approved. It's delivered for me on dates, it's delivered for me in the office, it's delivered for me on the dance floor. What can I say? Things happen when you wear an LBJ. I would go so far as to declare that every woman should have one in her life, and that is not something I propose lightly.

INTRODUCING CO-ORDS

A final option is "co-ords," a relatively new addition to the fashion line-up. Co-ords are a matching top and bottom, so not strictly speaking one-stop at all, but because they are in the same pattern—they usually are patterned—present like a one piece. The bottom half tends to be culottes—which look contemporary—though may also be a skirt or pants. Some clever brands produce a couple of alternatives.

Co-ords are particularly good if you are a different size on your top and bottom, or if you are long in the body but like the jumpsuit look. Co-ords also give you choices. The very one-stop-ness of the dress and the jumpsuit makes them harder—though far from impossible—to reinvent (their only downside). Whereas with co-ords you can dial down those patterned culottes with a jacket or sweater in a complementary neutral, or wear that look-at-me top with jeans or track pants at the weekend.

This can be a great way to extend the afterlife of an outfit that you bought for a special occasion but that you worry might be just a little too flamboyant for the rest of your life. Co-ords might add one extra element to that Wonder Woman spin, but I still think Diana Prince, Wonder Woman herself, would approve.

107

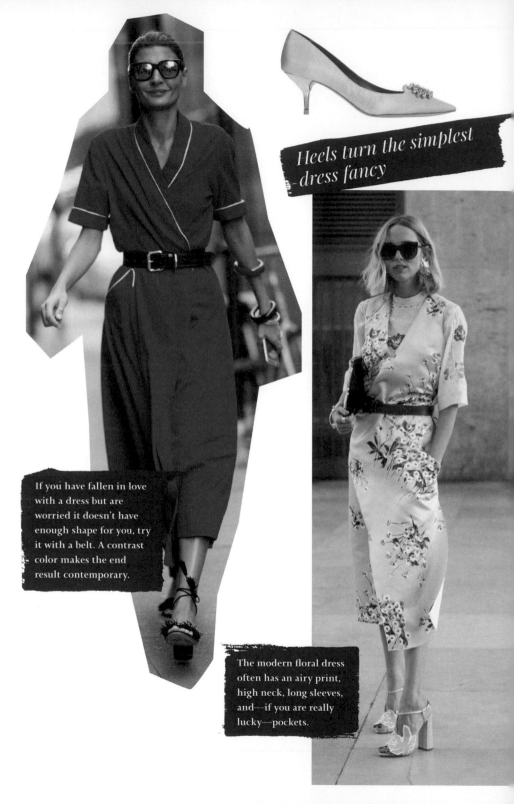

108

Heels turn the simplest dress fancy

If you have fallen in love with a dress but are worried it doesn't have enough shape for you, try it with a belt. A contrast color makes the end result contemporary.

The modern floral dress often has an airy print, high neck, long sleeves, and—if you are really lucky—pockets.

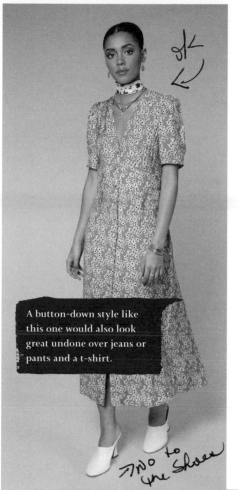

A button-down style like this one would also look great undone over jeans or pants and a t-shirt.

NOT JUST FOR PARTIES

There's a dress out there that will make every one of us look our best. That's why they're for everyday, not just special occasions. The right dress will smooth lines, highlight the good bits, and disguise the not-so-good. Plus a dress is unmess-upable (technical term), in that no mixing and matching is required. Buy right and it's all done for you. You can choose to keep things sleek and plain, or embrace what's becoming a real permatrend: the floral gown. Once seen as frumpy, it is now cool-girl, and works on all ages and sizes. Pick modernizing accessories, and wear with attitude.

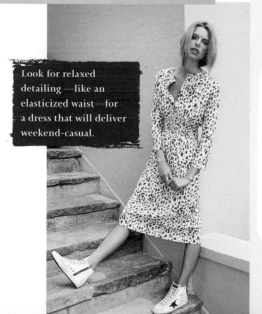

Look for relaxed detailing —like an elasticized waist—for a dress that will deliver weekend-casual.

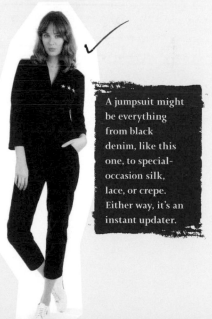

A jumpsuit might be everything from black denim, like this one, to special-occasion silk, lace, or crepe. Either way, it's an instant updater.

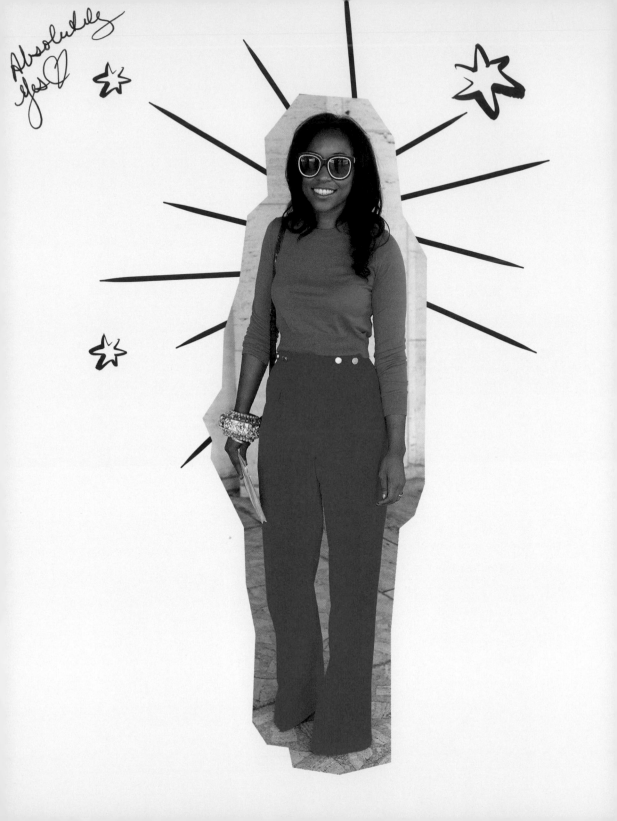

Absolutely
Yes ♡

7

21st-Century *Tweaks*

NEW-GENERATION LAYERING, PLUS MIXING-AND-NON-MATCHING

Looking modern is not just about what you wear, but how you wear it. So much has changed over the course of the last few decades concerning the lives women live. No surprise that the way we dress has changed in tandem.

It's comparatively easy to get your head around what's new when it comes to individual items of clothing, be it statement sneakers (yes, really) or power florals (ditto), even if it may still take you a while before you are prepared to dip your toe in the water and try them out yourself.

Much harder is to clock the subtle changes in the way people wear what they wear. And it can be harder still to attempt to pull off those shifts yourself. Yet if you get your head around the two big tweaks in contemporary dress codes, you will immediately modernize your look.

LAYER IT UP

The first is what I call "new-generation layering." I know that many of us still struggle with the idea of layering period, never mind any more recent incarnation. A friend who runs a high-street fashion brand tells me that the question his shopping advisors are asked most often by customers is, "How do I layer?"

So don't panic. You may not realize it but what you are doing pretty much every day of your life is layering. Coat over dress? Layering. Sweater over shirt? Layering. You can definitely already pull off the old-school variety.

When it comes to the new-gen incarnation, not only should you not panic, but you should also get ready to enjoy yourself. Because, once you have got the knack, it's a veritable *millefeuille* of fashion fun. You will soon relish doing it, and you will relish even more the way you look as a result.

Pleasingly, so will other people. New-gen layering is a matchless compliment-garnerer, because it makes you appear younger, cooler, and the opposite of try-hard. Indeed, don't be surprised if some of your friends start stealing your look.

That's how it started for me with new-gen layering. I still

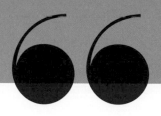

I like to improvise, as if I'm playing jazz. I usually have some sort of vision before I get started, and it's quick.

—IRIS APFEL

Find your friends

It can be helpful to take your fashion cues from stylish people whose path you cross every day. Friends, acquaintances, even people you just pass on the street. These are the women who have the potential to be not so much a style icon—with all the distance that suggests—but a style friend: someone who can be useful to you when it comes to finding your own way.

That's because these women—unlike movie stars and the like—are more likely to be living a life that's relevant to yours, with regard to everything from climate to what makes up their day-to-day. If you know someone, or meet them in the run of things, the content of their existence overlaps with yours. Look for people who have a similar body shape to yours. There's no point trying to steal a skinny minnie's look if you are curvy.

Also, if you see someone wearing something you admire, don't ever hesitate to tell them how much you like it, nor ask them where it's from. The best shoppers are never shy. I've lost track of the number of recommendations I've gotten everywhere from the supermarket to an art gallery. Nor is this only a practical matter. Making another woman feel good about herself, making her smile, is a small but significant way of strengthening the sisterhood. Let's admire each other, empower each other, and not just around the big things.

remember the day a decade or so ago when a front-row chum of mine began pairing items I considered anything but related.

First time around it was in the office, and she wore a tailored short-sleeved tunic—think a kind of buttonless jacket—layered over a silk blouse, topped off with some slim-cut black pants. She looked like she meant business—dressy and serious—but she also looked up to date. More than that, she looked original, and I would argue that standing out just enough in the office is a good thing. Original dresser, original thinker. Those are the kind of connections people make in their subconscious, whether they are aware of it or not. At work particularly, you are at least in part what you wear. (As well as lots of more important things besides, needless to say.)

A couple of weeks later, for a trip to the movies, my friend had turned that same tailored top casual by, this time, layering it over a long-sleeved tee, both stacked on top of a pair of classic straight-leg jeans. Hmmm, I thought to myself, she's onto something here. I need to get onto it quickly, too. I have been new-gen layering ever since.

It is about mixing different weights of material, and juxtaposing items that would once have been deemed incompatible.

HOW TO "NEW GEN" YOURSELF

You've probably got the general idea. In essence it is about mixing different weights of material, and juxtaposing items that would once have been deemed incompatible.

Like my friend—and these days me—you might choose to focus on your top half, and layer a long-sleeved tee or silk blouse under a short-sleeved or sleeveless sweater, blazer, or tailored tunic. I have another similarly chic friend who might take off her suit jacket to reveal two tees, a short-sleeved worn over a long-sleeved. Very cool. Even though the individual elements are classics, combined in this way they look instantly contemporary.

A default look among the fashion pack for the last couple of years has been a masculine tailored jacket undone over a feminine floaty dress. A double-breasted take is the favorite on the front row, a style which I know strikes fear into many women's hearts. A straight cut will work on small busts and straight figures. A fitted style can work on curvy and large-busted shapes. Try it. But if it's still adding too much bulk—again, your friend the full-length mirror will tell you—go for single-breasted.

Bear in mind that layering can be a great way to draw attention away from a long torso, or to add interest if you are tall. On the other hand, if you are petite, proceed with caution—too many layers may appear busy and/or shortening.

You might go head-to-toe, layering an unbuttoned softly draping floral summer dress over a black or white tee and trousers or jeans. Or that dress might be a wrap or kimono style. Or it might not be a dress at all, but a duster coat or silk robe. Bear in mind that your layers should be mostly soft, and mostly thin. Unless you are very slim, you don't want to add volume all over. Which is why you may also want on occasion to factor in a belt to give further definition.

Then you could add a shearling vest over the top, too. Or perhaps pair the vest with the same dress—if it is a dress— fastened up, and minus the underlayer. Or how about taking that vest and layering it under a trench or a wool overcoat for extra warmth, and for a glimmer of just-visible glamour? This is a version of what the fashion industry calls trans-seasonality, and which I call common sense: assembling outfits that can be built up or stripped down depending on the temperature of the day in question.

In case you haven't guessed already, I happen to think every woman should have a shearling vest in her possession. Not just because it is a one-stop route to the modernizing genius that is new-gen layering, but also because in terms of price-per-wear it will quickly prove itself to be one of your most parsimonious purchases.

Sure, a shearling vest isn't cheap up front, but if you play the long game, and I believe that when it comes to one's wardrobe that is what one should be doing nine times out of ten, it will end up costing you pennies every time you put it on. Why? Because you will just keep putting it on. Day after day, whatever that day promises.

I wear mine on the sofa. I wear it to weddings. I wear it everywhere in-between. It has repaid my initial investment countless times over. That said, if you still feel you can't stretch to such a sum check out the countless excellent faux options.

Or how about, if you are up for pushing the new-gen-layering envelope further, slipping a thin hoodie under a blazer? Sounds bonkers. Yet worn with a sleek pantsuit a hoodie provides a perfect storm of the cutting edge and the chic. Again, this delivers that original-dresser/original-thinker double whammy. Great if yours is the more open-minded variety of office.

MIXING-AND-NON-MATCHING

117

It also happens to be an example of my second 21st-century tweak, mixing-and-non-matching. Tailoring plus athleisure. What genre-busting! And genre-busting is another effortless way to update how you present to the world.

no absolutely no

In case you haven't guessed already, I happen to think every woman should have a shearling vest in her possession.

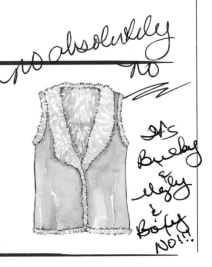

As Bulky Ugly & Boxy NO!!!

Seemingly incongruous couplings are proving to be a permatrend. From girly floral dresses with clunky macho ankle boots and/or a blazer, to a tuxedo jacket with jeans, to tailoring with sneakers. Then there are the countless individual items that do the genre-busting for you: statement sneakers; rhinestone-strewn denim; embroidery-covered sweatshirts, olive jackets, and cargo pants. The list is nigh on endless, and each item is a one-stop take on the theme of mixing-and-non-matching.

Trans-seasonality comes into play again, too. How about a big woolly sweater with silky skirt, woolly tights, and motorcycle boots for a January catch up with a girlfriend? Don't manage your next catch up until the summer? Ditch the sweater and the tights, and add in a tee. Or, given the unpredictability of modern weather, hang on to that sweater!

There's a further incarnation, namely the juxtaposing of colors, patterns, and prints in such a way as to once have been deemed akin to a crime against fashion. The street-stylers who get photographed outside the catwalk shows are past masters at this. Why? Because it's a way to dial up otherwise practical clothing. Even they don't like to look as if they are suffering for their art, and like to be able to walk, so they often wear functional individual pieces, then render them suitably look-at-me courtesy of mixing-and-non-matching. Iris Apfel is several decades older than most other street-stylers and out-mash-ups them all. "I like to improvise," she says, "as if I'm playing jazz. I usually have some sort of vision before I get started, and it's quick."

There's a further incarnation, namely the juxtaposing of color, patterns, and prints in such a way as to once have been deemed akin to a crime against fashion.

RAINBOW RULES

Let's take color first. There are two ways to approach it, and they both involve you getting your head around the color wheel (see p.81). Contrast hues that sing rather than clash tend to be opposites on the wheel: green and red; orange and blue; purple and yellow. That's option one. Option two is tone-on-tone combinations. That's what red and pink is. It used to be the ultimate no-no. Now it's practically *de rigueur* outside the shows. Violet and lilac is another one. A bright green with a pale green. It's fun once you start.

The stealth approach is to go for one majority hue, with a mere flash of something else. A pink pantsuit, for example, with a just-visible red underlayer. Then, should you not be in the mood to clash-match, you can dial down that pink pantsuit by wearing it with a white, cream, black, or navy underlayer instead. Not that a pink pantsuit can ever be dialed down that much, of course. Which is precisely what makes it so wonderful, but—for many of us—so terrifying.

THE PATTERN BOOK

Floral mash-ups, or pairing of different stripes, or spots, or both, are also par for the course these days. Striped shirt plus striped blazer plus striped skirt. That's not going to stop you running for the bus, or rather, in the case of the street-styler set, posing for the photographers who swarm outside each catwalk venue. But it is going to look fabulous enough, different enough, to get their attention in the first place.

Thing is, back in the real world, attempting the head-to-toe approach can go easily wrong. It's complicated—and expensive—to buy pieces that work together in this way. And even if you do pull it off, precisely because an outfit like this looks so distinctive, you may quickly tire of it. The simplest route is always to keep at least one part of your ensemble neutral. Striped shirt and blazer, maybe, but wear with jeans or black or navy pants, don't go full head-to-toe.

Start by pairing two more classic patterns: two contrast stripes, for example, or two checks. Much easier than attempting it with two florals. If you mix types of pattern—a stripe with a floral, say—pull things together by using the same color palette. A turquoise floral blouse layered over a turquoise checked pencil skirt could look fab. You might also want to think about giving new life to print by changing things up via the fabric it's delivered in. A traditionally "winter" print such as leopard or houndstooth looks ineffably modern rendered in silk. Or conversely how about a "summer" floral reincarnated as a luxurious wool coat? Whichever approach you go for, wear it with confidence, and with a smile. That makes pretty much everything look great.

Or buy a single piece that does the work for you. Buy a dress that splices two florals, rather than attempting to clash-match a blouse and skirt. Buy a shirt made of two different stripes. As mentioned before, you can bend the rules more quietly by mixing black and navy, a double-act that was once deemed unacceptable, yet is now verging on a dress code on the front row. Another stealth route is wearing gold and silver jewelry at one-and-the-same time. For me these are the simplest real-world routes to channeling the genre-busting zeitgeist.

So many of us have an objection hard wired in our brains to black and navy, and to silver and gold, that it can again help to start with a single piece that breaks the rules for us. Perhaps a black crepe dress with a navy trim, or a navy blouse with black detailing.

When it comes to jewelry, a classic bracelet watch that combines both metals is a great way to get the ball rolling. But now there are countless other baubles that combine the two. Once you have built up your confidence you can channel the magpie approach, stockpiling gossamer contrast pieces at the neck, wrists, and fingers so that they somehow, due to their fairylike dimensions, come together as a sum that's greater than its parts.

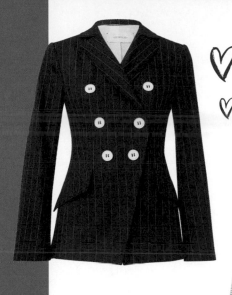

yes Absolutely

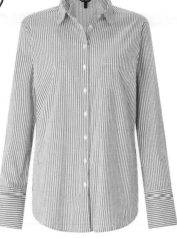

STRIPED JACKET

STRIPED SHIRT

NEUTRAL PANTS

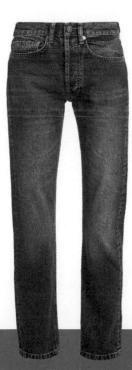

... *when you can wear two different ones? Or even, if you are feeling very brave, three? I love this outfit. It looks put-together yet casual. It feels classic yet— thanks to those contrast stripes— up to date.*

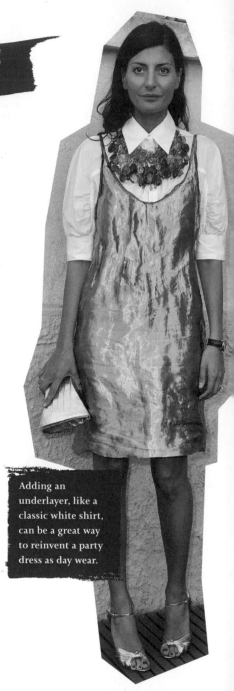

Buy ready-mixed gold and silver

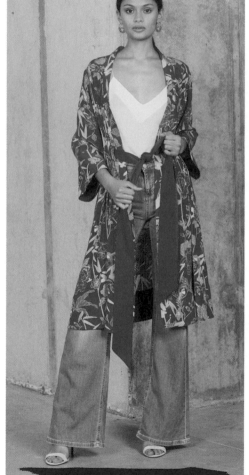

Pair an undone kimono—or button-down or wrap dress—over jeans and a tee for the ultimate in contemporary clash-matches.

Adding an underlayer, like a classic white shirt, can be a great way to reinvent a party dress as day wear.

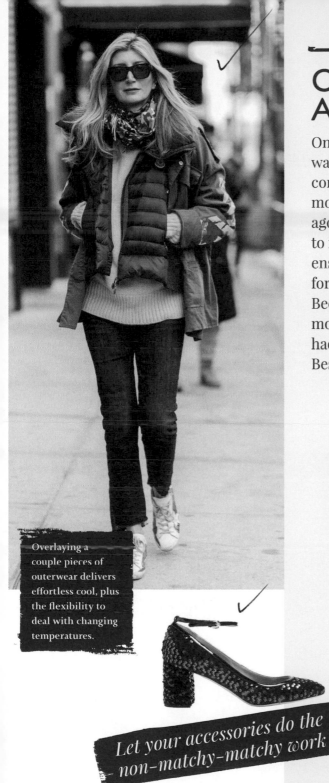

OPPOSITES ATTRACT

One of the biggest shifts in the way the fashion-forward dress: to conjure up an outfit from two or more items that, only a few years ago, it would've been impossible to imagine as part of the same ensemble. It can be intimidating for the rest of us. So why bother? Because it will make you look modern, often using pieces you've had in your wardrobe for years. Besides, it's not as hard as it looks.

Sharp tailoring spliced with street wear adds up to a contemporary look, whatever your age.

Overlaying a couple pieces of outerwear delivers effortless cool, plus the flexibility to deal with changing temperatures.

Let your accessories do the non-matchy-matchy work

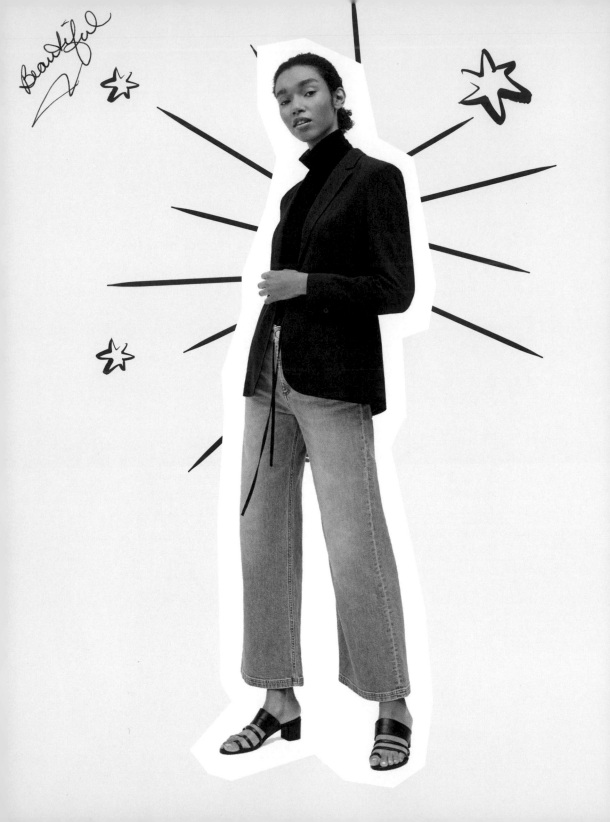

8

Sustainable
Fashion

WHAT IT REALLY MEANS,
HOW TO PULL IT OFF

How to become a better fashion consumer? It's now almost as common a conversation among the front row as where to find the perfect jeans. And the answer is, if anything, even less straightforward, even more open to interpretation.

Most of us are trying to figure out how to be better consumers, be it of fashion, food, fuel, or anything else you care to mention. And those of us who aren't should be. A true happy-ever-after wardrobe isn't just about you, but about our planet, our children's planet.

How to love that planet, as well as to love fashion? The easy part of the equation is that we need to buy less, which is why learning how to buy better is so important. What better means when it comes to flattering your body, working with your lifestyle, and making you feel like the best possible version of you, is comparatively simple. What better means in terms of cost to the environment and impact on workers in the production chain is considerably trickier.

One thing that's clear is that we need to be prepared to spend a little more. It's not that you need to have money to look chic. Indeed, financial abundance often leads to a scattered approach to clothes buying, which in turn results in a wardrobe that at best lacks focus, and at worst is out of control. "I see a lot of women who don't have money, who don't spend, and they look chic beyond," observes the designer Carolina Herrera. "And I see a lot of women who spend a lot of money, who buy everything they see, and don't look good."

But the fact is that the rise of so-called fast fashion has given us a false sense of the true cost of the production process of, say, a jacket. If the people who produce that jacket are properly paid, and if the environment doesn't pay the price either, it may cost more than many of us are currently prepared to spend. A friend who worked as a buyer for a budget brand said that her job became impossible, as margins were ever more squeezed to keep costs down. She would be instructed to tell a manufacturer that they had to produce a piece for a certain price while at the same time

"

My mother
taught me that
style is about
attitude. It has
nothing to do
with money.

—IRIS APFEL

guaranteeing it was ethical. Said manufacturer would reply that it could be done, but only if someone paid the price of that cost-cutting, and that someone would always be the workers and Mother Earth. My friend has since left her job.

FROM FAST TO SLOW FASHION

It's worth noting what a recent phenomenon fast fashion is. The term was only coined in 1989 to describe Zara's "quick response" model. This concept had first been introduced earlier in that same decade by the American clothing industry, which had in turn borrowed it from the Japanese car industry. Its original intent was to improve efficiencies in manufacturing and supply chains. It did that. But it also turned us all into trend junkies.

Our mothers and grandmothers—even the most clothes addicted among them—bought in a way that was measured, and with a view to the long term. Our shopping habits would be unrecognizable to them. Almost half of Chinese consumers now buy more than they can afford, with around 40 percent qualifying as excessive shoppers. Can we re-learn how to shop as our predecessors did? Can we shake off our fast-fashion addiction?

One consideration that might help us go cold turkey: has all of this consuming made us any more stylish? Absolutely not. Many of us have actually lost our way as a result. We've developed a kind of trends-blindness—think snow-blindness but a lot more expensive—which means that, though we may buy more than we used to, we tend not to wear most of it.

Our wardrobes may be bulging but we—I—default to a smaller capsule iteration eked out from around its edges. While we may be endlessly tempted into buying the kind of fantastical fashion that

Has all this consuming actually made us any more stylish? Absolutely not.

Sarah Jessica Parker used to wear in *Sex and the City*, in practice—if we are lucky; if we are getting it right—we default to the edited timeless chic she now wears in *Divorce*. (There's a metaphor in there somewhere!) We tend to feel happier if we manage to enact just a little school-of-Marie-Kondo thinking and throw out— sorry, upcycle—the things we don't wear so we can eyeball the things we do.

"Fashion has always been about novelty," says Dilys Williams, from the London College of Fashion's Centre for Sustainable Fashion. But it didn't necessarily used to be about more. "We used to be more adaptive. There used to be less through-put." In other words, we would keep things longer and make them work harder for us: mixing-and-matching; retooling an old item to look new; look-lifting by way of small add-ons (see Chapter 14). And, as Williams continues, though we may buy far more than our forebears, "We don't look any more stylish or distinctive than people used to."

These days sustainable fashion doesn't need to appear worthy: it can look like, well, fashion. Take the va-va-voom Calvin Klein dress that the actress Emma Watson wore to the Met Gala in 2016 as part of the so-called Green Carpet Challenge. It was a million miles from the plastic bottles it started life as. Proof positive that there is such a thing as green-hot. Indeed, pretty much whatever your heart desires is now available in a planet-friendly incarnation if you buy from the right brands. You could glam it up in a sequinned skirt, biker jacket, and heels and still be ticking all the right boxes.

NATURAL ISN'T ALWAYS BEST

But what does sustainable fashion mean exactly? Even the lexicon can be confusing. First it was green. Then it was eco. Now it's sustainable. These terms are synonymous, but also nebulous. "How do you measure sustainability? Where does it start? Where does it stop?" asks Rebecca Earley of the Centre for Circular Design, part of the University of the Arts London. "Every aspect of a textile, of the production of a garment, has complexities."

Many of the layperson's assumptions about what is or isn't good for the planet can be misguided. I always thought natural fibers were preferable. Yet cotton, for example, is a voracious consumer of water, especially in climates to which it is not suited, such as China's—currently the second-biggest global producer. Recycled polyester, on the other hand, a by-product of the petrochemical industry, gets the thumbs up from Earley. Similarly, man-made Tencel®, which, like all forms of viscose, is plant-based and therefore neither truly synthetic nor truly natural, "is going to solve a lot of problems in the future." Yep. This stuff is a head spin.

It's these complexities that go a long way toward explaining why legislative change is coming at such a slow pace around the world. The buzzword for the future, Earley tells me, is "circular." "It's measurable," she says. "You either close the loop or you don't. This is what is going to give us a framework going forward. Using so-called Life Cycle Analysis [LCA], we can determine that, say, one dress is 40 percent better than another."

It also matters what happens to a garment after it's bought. We wash our clothes too often. One of the biggest environmental impacts of the average cotton t-shirt, according to Earley, will come via our over-laundering. We also throw clothes away too readily. Buying less is, again, part of the solution here. But it's also about looking after what we have: de-pilling our sweaters and invisible-mending the holes in our clothes.

One of the biggest environmental impacts of the average cotton t-shirt will come via our over-laundering.

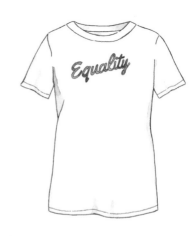

Putting on the pressure

We need to ask questions of the brands we buy clothes from, and to become as informed as we can be about what presents a bad purchasing choice vs a good one or an even better one. Thankfully, there are some key pressure groups than can help us with this, each of them targeting different aspects of sustainability.

The Ellen MacArthur Foundation, for example, is focused on sustainability in the most literal sense, demanding that companies recycle and buy back more, and that we—the consumer—buy less and keep it longer.

Slaveryfootprint.org campaigns against modern-day slavery. You can take its excellent online survey to find out, in the words of the website, "how many slaves are working for you." Fascinating and terrifying.

Then there's the Sustainable Apparel Coalition, number-cruncher extraordinaire: an industry-led initiative that draws on scientific evidence to determine the environmental impact of particular materials. It also brings together direct competitors such as Nike and Adidas to collaborate on improving their practices.

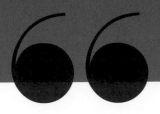

Some think it's all about consumers changing their wicked ways, others that it's businesses that are doing the harm. In practice it's both.

—REBECCA EARLEY

CHANGING OUR APPROACH

Dilys Williams believes that the initial legislative changes will focus on "specific issues." First up, like as not, will be laws to deal with "microfibers that go back into the water system, and big global issues like water stress." (By 2030 global demand for water will outstrip supply.) In the meantime, she continues, "we don't need legislation to tell us what good fashion is. It's about a culture change."

Can we alter our habits? Research would suggest that millennials already are, with 66 percent willing to spend more on brands that are sustainable, according to *The State of Fashion 2018* report by the Business of Fashion and McKinsey. But the culture change has to be corporate, too. "Some think it's all about consumers changing their wicked ways," says Rebecca Earley, "others that it's businesses that do the harm. In practice it's both."

On this Williams expresses cautious optimism. "The big guys know legislation is coming. They are already sourcing from places with scarcity of water and other resources. They know that they can't continue as they are." Some brands have enlightened leadership. Some are acting from more immediate self-interest, responding not only to consumer interest but also to economic exigencies. "If you recycle your materials, you cut your costs," says Earley.

The luxury group Kering—home to Gucci and Alexander McQueen—gets a gold star for its introduction of a tool called the Environmental Profit & Loss Account, which it now publishes in its annual report, and which reveals the cost to nature of its fashion production in that year. Meanwhile, fast-fashion behemoths such as H&M and Mango have sustainable collections.

STEP BY STEP

Is it hypocrisy that mega-brands—be they high street or luxury—should be flying the sustainability flag from their flagpoles while at the same time tempting us to spend, spend, spend? Of course. Yet interestingly the experts seem to see that hypocrisy as a

133

necessary one. "No business can turn around overnight," says Williams. "By starting to transform sections of their company they can trial ways to make more wholesale changes." (And give us a means to vote with our wallets.) "H&M, for example, is doing some big work. They are very serious about change. And Kering is really leading the way."

For now there is no single brand or website that has all the answers, but there are growing numbers that will help you feel as good about the provenance of what you are buying as about how it makes you look. Search out those who are clear about their statement of intent, and who give detailed information on the provenance of everything they sell.

Here is my Top 20 of those who are leading the way. Go forth and shop, but only if you really think you need to.

1

G-STAR RAW
Their Raw for the Planet denim is made with 98 percent recycled water.

2

EILEEN FISHER
A transparent and trailblazing American label. Its Renew collection resells or retools items sent in by customers.

3

H&M CONSCIOUS
Sustainable fabric innovation is one focus in this fashion-forward annual collection.

4

GATHER & SEE
Some dialed-down basics, some statement pieces, from a range of cool, little known brands. What's not to like?

5

NINETY PERCENT
A new sustainable British leisure wear brand; 90 percent of its profits are donated to charity.

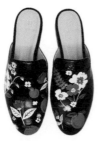

6

MAISON DE MODE
A favorite with movie stars who like their carpet to be green not red.

7
FONNESBECH
A Scandinavian game changer that delivers a tight edit on a minimalist aesthetic.

8
MANGO COMMITTED
This annual collection from the fast-fashion behemoth is at the forefront of its forays into sustainability.

9
KITX
A high-end Australian label with rigorous sustainability standards, and a just-zeitgeist-enough feel.

10
POSITIVE LUXURY
This website has a Sustainability Council that includes high-profile figures like Jonathon Porritt.

11
MAIYET
A stealth-wealth American brand that partners with artisans from around the world.

12
RÊVE EN VERT
Another celebrity favorite that's as strong at off-duty as on-carpet brands.

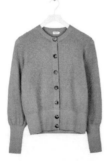

13
FILIPPA K
This top sustainability brand will treat or repair any garment as part of its "10 Years of Care" program.

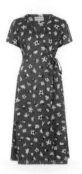

14
THEORY
This American label's 2.0 Collection has sustainability at its core, with refreshed-classic styling that will serve you 24/7.

15
PEOPLE TREE
This multi-award-winning website launched 26 years ago, and still offers a wide range of sustainable, affordable fashion.

16
WE ARE THOUGHT
An Australian brand that delivers affordable, practical clothes leavened by some great prints.

17
STELLA MCCARTNEY
A trailblazing British luxury brand, which uses recycled and sustainable materials.

18
ANTIBAD
A wide range of price points, but a singularity of focus, this website is particularly good on affordable bags and shoes.

19
THE ACEY
Founded in 2014 by fashion pro Holly Ellenby who set out to find "innovative, conscious" brands.

20
EDUN
A luxury label that delivers discreet style with a twist.

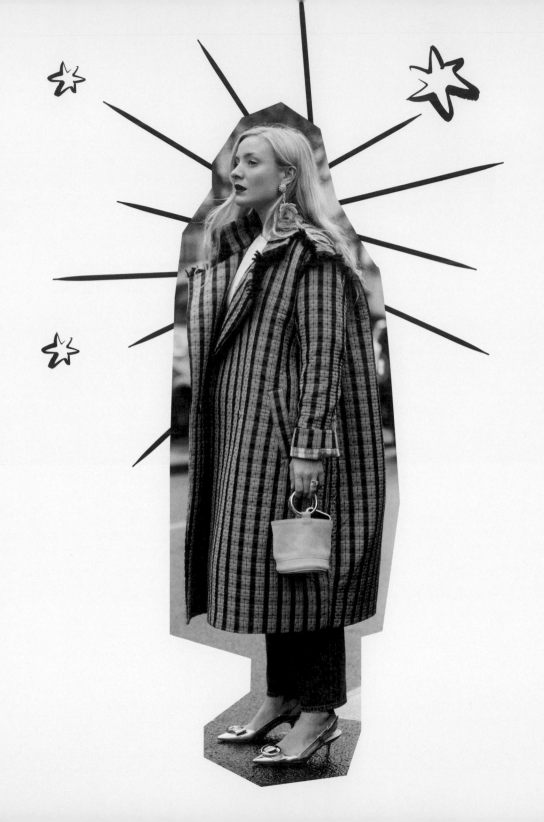

9

Fancy
Footwork

SHOES, GLORIOUS SHOES

As many of us know instinctively, often addictively, shoes are so much more than a finishing touch. Like nothing else—and I mean nothing—what you wear on your feet can transform your look.

If you peruse old family photographs from a few decades ago and examine the women, I wager it will be their shoes more than anything that will reveal them to be of an era different than our own.

Fashion is in the recycling game, now more than ever. You could walk into a store today and buy a dress that might be confused with one from the 1940s. But a pair of shoes? No. Even those that declare themselves to be retro in style will have been tweaked to update them.

So if you have been buying shoes on repeat for years, or indeed not buying any at all—unlikely, I imagine—stop. You may well need to rethink. "If you want to modernize your look, and you can only spend money on one thing," says the personal shopper Anna Berkeley, "shoes are key. They can ruin an outfit in a nanosecond." And, by the same token, reinvent it. The shoe designer Christian Louboutin believes this is why shoes have become one of the defining fashion items of our age. "Fashion has become so standardized," he told me recently, "that it's the details that make the difference. The finishing touches. The jewelry but, above all, the shoes."

Shopping for shoes should be one of the most fun, least problematic fashion transactions. That's why so many of us are like a proto–Imelda Marcos. (Actually wearing them can, alas, be a different matter, as proven by the blisters we have all endured at some point in our lives.) Though you may need to tweak what you buy slightly, you will still enjoy the process, promise.

WHAT'S MODERN?

A few things to get your head around in terms of what looks current. There's a chunkiness, even a clunkiness that would have been unimaginable only a few years ago. (This isn't for everyone. More anon.) Then there's the influence of athleisure (see Chapter 11). Sneakers are everywhere, and often so pimped as to appear a

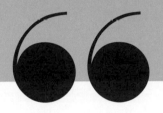

When I started shoes were only black and brown, sometimes white, sometimes red. Bags, too. I was working during the period when accessories became fashion items."

—MARIA GRAZIA CHIURI

world apart from their track-and-field origins. When is a sneaker not a sneaker? Perhaps when it is encrusted with sequin flowers and costs a three-figure sum that starts with a seven. Sneakers have also hybridized with other types of shoes, with varying degrees of success: there are platform sandals with sneaker soles, sneakers with wedge heels, and boots with sports-ready strapping.

The ubiquity of the sneaker can be linked to all those elements that have prompted the rise of athleisure more generally. Comfort is part of it. The shoes we wear to the office each day, to the playground, to shop, to meet friends for dinner—often all four—need to be friend, not foe.

The shoes we wear to the office each day, to the playground, to shop, to meet friends for dinner—often all four— need to be friend, not foe.

142

THE RISE OF THE FLAT

Women used to work long hours in the home. They had plenty to worry about—you imagine life without a washing machine—but getting through the day in heels wasn't one of them. They wore slippers, or the hard-soled version known as house shoes; far from alluring but super-comfortable. When they first went out to work in offices, they attempted to do it in heels. Now, finally, more and more of us are wearing flats, or lower heels, heels that—dare I say it—are comfortable. But we need to look great. We need a house shoe that looks like an office shoe, in other words. We need to be stealth-shod.

Hence the rise of the flat, so to speak. Flat shoes are—surprise, surprise—easier to get through the day in than heels. They are the sensible option for those of us whose professional life dictates that we should look dressier than sneakers permit, sequinned or otherwise. But they don't have to be boring any more.

Because that is the other change in footwear, a change that has come about precisely because we are demanding practicality. How to stop a practical shoe looking dull? By lavishing attention on it via embellishment. There are now flat shoes at every price so intricately adorned as to have passed muster at the court of the Sun King.

When it comes to flats, there's also another kind of embellishment. A heel. Hang on a minute, I am not going mad. It's a heel so tiny that it barely merits the name, at most 1¾in, often less. The fashion industry calls it the nano-heel. I call it the kit heel, not just because it's smaller than the classic kitten, but because it is also more serviceable; part of a proper uniform designed to serve you 24/7, along with your cross-body bag (see p.91) and a power piece or two. Kit heels are the ultimate addition to your arsenal if you are a heel lover and sole-ache loather. (And everyone is the latter.)

IT'S ALL IN THE DETAIL

Three other styling tweaks that keep on running. A low-cut front which reveals toe cleavage (yes, it's a thing). Cone heels—a fresh take on the user-friendly mid-heel. And footbed or fussbett sandals: think orthopaedic footwear turned chic. Not for everyone, but a great way to add cool.

Other changes? That shoes can be every color under the sun: white pumps and white or red ankle boots, for example, are both heading toward permatrend status. Scarlet boots can transform a pantsuit—be it in a neutral or a brighter hue—into something special. Push it further again with some matching earrings.

It didn't used to be this way. Maria Grazia Chiuri, now head design honcho at Dior, started her career in accessories. "The biggest revolution in fashion in the last twenty years has been in accessories, not in fashion. When I started shoes were only black and

There are now flat shoes at every price so intricately adorned as to have passed muster at the court of the Sun King.

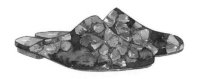

brown, sometimes white, sometimes red. Bags, too. I was working during the period when accessories became fashion items."

This is why shoes have more transformative power than ever before. A classic kitten heel can look altogether new in neon orange, for example, and in turn can render a navy dress altogether new-looking, too.

Even affordable shoes now come in materials that would once have been as impossibly luxurious. Patent is verging on old hat. How about velvet, satin, and raffia? I am not going to pretend to you that these are the most practical choices, but if you buy a reasonably priced iteration, and wear with care, they can be a great way to freshen an outfit. What unites this new-generation footwear is a sense of fun, of frivolity, albeit with that backbone of wearability. Good news! And you don't have to spend large amounts of money.

THE POWER BOOT

The biggest permatrend is those mid-heel ankle boots, as worn with dresses and skirts by the cool-girl fraternity in the worlds of tech and media. These are a one-stop—or, to be precise, two-stop—way to change up a look, because they add edge. A floral dress that might look girly worn with kitten heels looks punchy worn with ankle boots. That's why I have christened them the power boot. And, of course, they are easy to walk in thanks to the height of the heel, usually either a chunky style or a kitten. Plus there's the fact that they are securely on your feet. No accidentally sliding out of your power boots.

"

A floral dress that might look girly worn with kitten heels looks punchy worn with ankle boots.

KEEP IT CONTEMPORARY

You can still buy classic styles, but they should only be straight-down-the-line iterations if you are one of those people who is so intrinsically hip that everything you put on turns from frumpy to fabulous. You are probably skinny, you are probably young, and you definitely boast such a finely-honed fashion skill-set as to have a PhD in vintage shopping at the very least. You can wear the exact same loafers your mother wore years ago and look cool.

The rest of us will look like librarians. The rest of us need classics with a tweak. Perhaps a loafer with a pointed toe, or in a new-gen bright or metallic, or just that bit more chunky than it would once have been. Perhaps an emerald satin kitten heel. Perhaps a brogue with a sneaker sole, or in a gorgeous suede. Perhaps a pump with a cone heel.

Yes, you can still wear heels. Just make sure they are a height you can manage, even—especially—for a special event. "Never ever wear heels you can't walk in," says red-carpet stylist Rebecca Corbin-Murray. It's one of her key rules. She's right. There is no more definitive way to date your look then to wear shoes that hobble you. Thankfully there's no need to any more. Much of what's in the stores is a world away from those crippling high pumps worn by an earlier generation of women, and that television dramas insist on pretending we still wear even when we are in our kitchens today.

Just make sure that, whether you choose heels or flats, you change it up style-wise. Honestly. Then you will be changed up, too. And the more classical your taste when it comes to the rest of your attire the more this matters. Timeless tailoring looks up to date with sneakers, and it's hard to go wrong with a pair of those front-row favorites Adidas Stan Smiths. An ever-after LBD is transformed by some velvet platform sandals or some prettily embellished kitten heels.

FINDING THE SHOE THAT TRULY FITS

So how to find what works for you? It's not just a question of taste. It's also about what flatters your particular feet and your particular height and frame. If you are perfectly in proportion, medium in every way, then that's fine, but few of us are. If you are petite, you

145

The nitty-gritty

FRAME SIZE

LARGE FRAMED?
Look for thick heels and chunky platforms.
Avoid anything that bisects you horizontally, ankle straps (crossover straps, however, are universally flattering), and power boots, unless they are cut low enough to showcase the ankle.

SMALL FRAMED?
Look for dainty shoes. Slim kitten heels, stilettos, the most lithe of wedges.

MEDIUM FRAMED?
Look for surprise, surprise—something in the middle. Kitten heels, medium wedges, slim blocks, or flatforms.

FOOT SIZE

LARGE FEET?
Look for pretty detailing, rounded or square toe.
Avoid a low cut.

SMALL FEET?
Look for pointed toes and a low-cut front that will show off maximum flesh.
Avoid styles that are too fussy.

WIDE FEET?
Look for dark colors, plain styles, pointed toes, a soupçon of toe cleavage.

LARGE AND WIDE FEET?
Look for a softer-pointed or v-shape toe and diagonal straps and detailing. Wearing pants slightly long can provide another distraction.

NARROW FEET?
Look for horizontal details that will appear to widen the foot. Make sure heels and straps are kept slim, too.
Avoid long, pointed, Rip van Winkle toes.

don't want to look like a Will' o' the Wisp. If you are a bigger build you don't want to look bigger still.

It would also make sense to finesse your way to feet that fit the rest of you: to make large feet appear smaller, small feet larger, wide feet narrower, narrow feet wider. Yes, shoes can do all that for you, and more (see left).

I know, right? I bet you have never considered all of this before. But it's obvious when you think about it. Of course the same pair of shoes is going to look different on different people; what works wonders for one person can be disastrous for someone else, depending on body type. Think of Cinderella's glass slipper. Great for her. Not so good for the Ugly Step-Sisters.

PUT YOUR BEST FEET FORWARD

And what of the feet themselves? What about those long-suffering oft-overlooked heroines that take us places, day after day, decade after decade. Don't forget about them, and, more particularly, don't let your love of shoes end up hurting the feet that are supposed to last you a lifetime.

One of my grandmothers had bunions. My mother has been edging toward them, too. I could tell that my feet were just a couple of decades behind hers. Then I discovered silicon toe spacers, rather like those you wear when you have a pedicure, except that these don't inhibit you walking around, and can even be worn inside slippers. They were designed by a sports podiatrist with a view to giving us back the toes we have when we are born but which many of us—particularly shoe junkies such as myself— lose as we age. Suffice it to say there is nothing scarier than when a group of front-row women unveil their fashion-scarred feet. We have the feet of trolls.

Or at least I did have. Now, my toes are well on the way to become straight and separated again. Wear toe spacers for half an hour a day—or longer—and gradually your feet will start to transform. It seems a magical process. But it's brilliantly real. And leaves your feet in better shape to wear the shoes of your dreams.

148

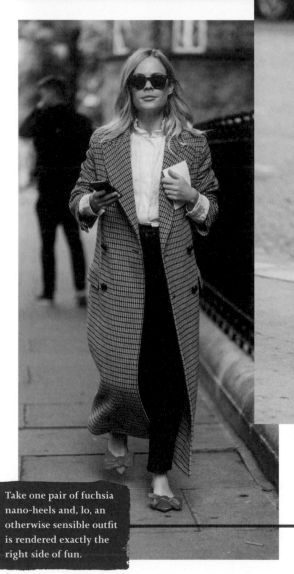

Look for flats with attitude

Platform sandals—which don't need to be as chunky as this style—make you seem taller with minimal heel height to negotiate.

Take one pair of fuchsia nano-heels and, lo, an otherwise sensible outfit is rendered exactly the right side of fun.

THE FOOTWEAR FULL MONTY

Gorgeousness plus comfort. At last there are shoes out there that deliver both. Ours is a footwear golden age, not least because so many of even the most practical styles come in blinged-out disguise, from metallic brocade to diamanté adornment. Bliss!

Power boots are here to stay. Why? Because they are as practical as it gets. And make everything appear modern.

A must whatever your age

Classic yet contemporary

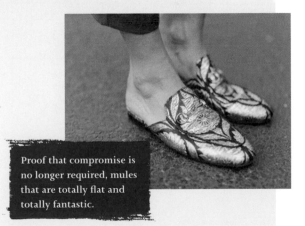

Proof that compromise is no longer required, mules that are totally flat and totally fantastic.

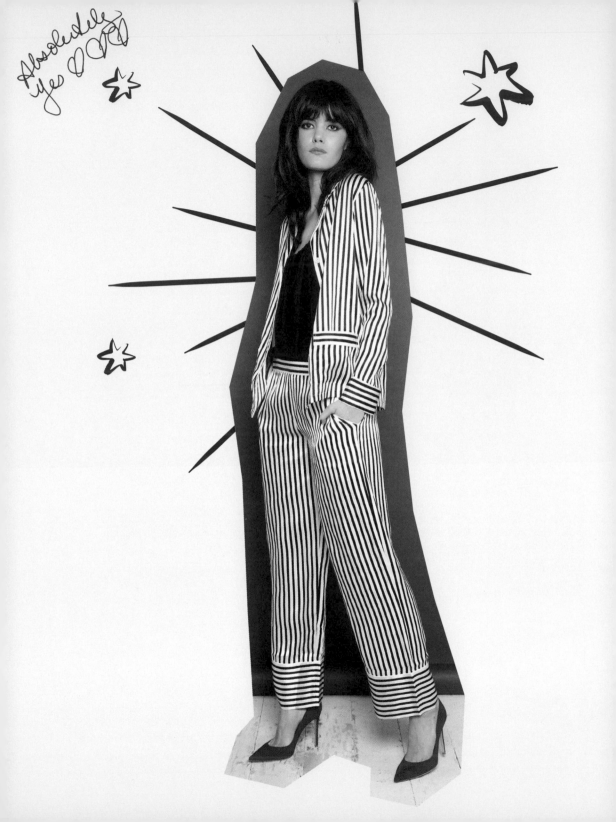

10

Flourish
Dressing

THE GAME-CHANGER PIECES THAT WILL TRANSFORM YOUR LOOK

Head to toe can be hard, especially when it comes to separates. Figuring out what goes with what can seem like one question too many in the morning. That's why so many of us default to a wardrobe dominated by a single neutral, usually black. And there is nothing wrong with black, if you've bought cannily—with an eye to quality and detail.

But cannier still is to use that blank—blanck?—canvas as a background to something special, a game-changer item that is going to transform the way you look, and probably the way you feel. It will usually entail color, or pattern, or both. If it doesn't then it will have to have detail so in-your-face as to class it as something else altogether, or be made in a fabric with such an interesting texture as to be a talking point in and of itself.

A black jacket, for example, turns game changer only when it has, say, military buttoning the likes of which hasn't been seen since a Russian hussar, or is rendered in an elaborate brocade, or— even better—encompasses both. And even then, a grandstanding soldier would favor red, or perhaps turquoise, so why shouldn't you? Two or three power pieces in a wardrobe are enough to alchemize a closet full of workhorse items into a whole that expresses your individuality. This is what will make you stand out, make you stylish, with minimal effort.

"Clothes are great fun, an exercise in creativity," says Iris Apfel. So let's enjoy them, express ourselves via them. But let's not forget what a serious business getting dressed is, too. "You never realize how much of your background is sewn into the lining of your clothes," wrote Tom Wolfe in *Bonfire of the Vanities*.

If you are clever you can "sew" whatever story you like about yourself via your clothes. Sew it with a flourish, what's more, and you get yourself noticed. Wolfe knew that. He loved an attention-grabbing white suit, the ultimate in flourish dressing. So, too, did that other great man of American letters, Mark Twain. "Little by little I hope to get together courage enough to wear white clothes all through the winter, in New York," the creator of *Huckleberry Finn* once wrote. If flourish dressing made sense to Twain and Wolfe,

"

Clothes are great fun, an exercise in creativity.

—IRIS APFEL

Gorgeous

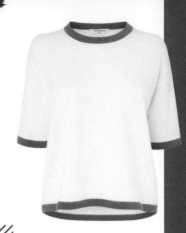

Pajamas have become a fashion-pack favorite, but not usually worn together. Pair the trousers with a neutral top—a t-shirt when it's hot, a sweater when it's cold. Keep it dialed down on your feet, too.

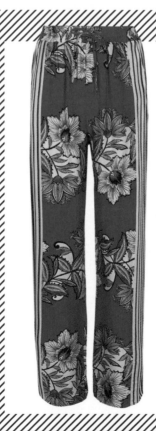

PLAIN TOP

SILK PAJAMA BOTTOMS

SIMPLE SHOES

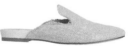

both the very opposite of flibbertigibbets, it should make sense to you.

That hot-hued jacket will render a workaday skirt or trousers away-day fabulous, while not compromising on functionality. A pair of patterned silk pajama bottoms will, when twinned with a plain t-shirt, make you look ready to go out on the town and party. Or, then again, to stay in for the most glamorous iteration imaginable of a night on the sofa. Or perhaps both—pretty much my perfect evening come to think of it: fun and games followed by r and r. An embroidered pencil skirt will, when matched with a school-uniform-style v-neck sweater, turn you into the coolest person at brunch, in the office, pretty much anywhere.

POWER PIECES *change things up: Great Jkt pants / scarf*

I call them power pieces, such is their capacity to change things up. I also call them passion pieces. Because clothes about which

Really love your Passion Pieces

you feel passionate will empower you. It's that easy. And they are easy to wear, too, because the whole point of flourish dressing is to keep everything else pared back.

It should go without saying that whatever it is that defines the item as a passion piece—be it color, pattern, texture, bold-facing detailing— you need to love it; really,

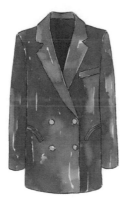

> **That hot-hued jacket will render a workaday skirt or trousers away-day fabulous, while not compromising on functionality.**

really love it. A passion piece is a sartorial smile, for you and for others who see you wearing it.

And they will see you wearing it. Because passion pieces are designed to draw attention to you. Which is, I promise, a good thing. Some of you may not agree with me on this one initially. Some of you may want your clothes to let you pass unnoticed. You shouldn't. And besides, don't kid yourself that you ever passed unnoticed, whatever you are or aren't wearing. Invisible clothes get you noticed for your invisibility. In other words, you get noticed then dismissed, a lose-lose situation if ever there was one. "In order to be irreplaceable one must always be different," is how Coco Chanel once put it.

But let's drill down into the precise nature of that noticing. What conclusions do you want people to draw about you from what you wear? Imagine yourself in a room full of strangers. What is the first word you would like to come into the mind of everyone who sees you before you exchange a sentence? It is revealing to think about what that word might be. When you have figured it out, it should inform the way you shop. Start to dress more visibly and, little by little, I promise you will come to enjoy it.

Perhaps that word is "chic." Perhaps it's "cool" or "effortless." Perhaps it's "creative." Perhaps it's "clever." And does that word change depending on the day at hand, or the event in question? For me that word is always "interesting." I want the way I look to make people think I have things to say. Clothes can do that for you. You just have to make sure to follow through with the chat.

Start to dress more visibly and, little by little, I promise you will come to enjoy it.

How I choose to look interesting may vary depending on whether I have an important meeting or a dinner with friends, and there may be other words that come into play, too, but for me the key word remains the same. Your chosen power pieces should embody that word or words.

DRESSING PHENOMENALLY

Beautiful

Maya Angelou was celebrated for what she did with language. But

156

Unforgettable

she used one of her most well-loved poems to acknowledge where her finely developed sense of style had got her. In "Phenomenal Woman" (1978) she writes:

> "Pretty women wonder where my secret lies.
> I'm not cute or built to suit a fashion model's size
> But when I start to tell them
> They think I am telling lies."

She goes on to name-check

> "the grace of my style …
> I don't shout or jump about
> Or have to talk real loud.
> When you see me passing,
> It ought to make you proud.
> I say,
> it's in the click of my heels,
> The bend of my hair
> the palm of my hand,
> The need for my care.
> 'Cause I'm a woman
> Phenomenally.
> Phenomenal woman,
> That's me."

Angelou dressed to be seen; to be admired. That didn't invalidate her formidable intellectual heft. Virginia Woolf—another heavy hitter—talked of "frock consciousness." For me there's a significant duality to the phrase. It's not only about recognizing the importance of what you wear, but also about determining how what you wear imprints upon your consciousness, and on other people's, and ensuring that it serves you well. Phenomenally, even.

what you wear imprints upon your consciousness & others

THE RIGHT FLOURISHES FOR YOU

Many of us are afraid of color and pattern. Don't be. Find what chimes for you, with you, and both can become a source of joy. You will come to pity men for the limited way in which most of them feel they can wear either, if they wear them at all.

In terms of pattern, the key is to look for a scale that works with your frame. Your wrist measurement will indicate whether you are small, medium, or large framed (see p.32). Pick a scale of pattern that echoes your frame size—large for large, medium for medium, small for (you guessed it) small. That's how to avoid looking on the one hand vast, on the other hand swamped.

Pick the right patterned piece and it will help you not just by changing your game, but by changing your shape. If your shape is angular go for angular prints: checks and stripes; hard-edged geometrics. If you're rounded, choose—yep—rounded patterns: fluid florals; scrolls and swirls; laciness and watery prints of all varieties. If you are interjacent—somewhere between the two—you should go for similarly halfway-house options: softened checks; more linear florals; animal print.

As for color, ignore trends, not least because there is now pretty much every hue on the catwalk every season. Instead examine your complexion. If you class as "warm"—with pink undertones and green veins—then you will look best in warmer tones like yellows and oranges. If yours is a cooler complexion—with yellow or green undertones and blue/purple veins—then you will suit cooler blues and purples. If you are a neutral—ashen or gray undertones; indeterminate vein color—you have freer rein (see p.79).

It's a good idea to get used to using that Carolina-Herrera-

Power pieces wave a flag not only generally, but also in a focused way, leading the eye to the section of the body that has been thus garbed.

If your top half is larger than your lower—if you are an inverted triangle, or a variation on the theme thereof— focus the flourishing on skirts and trousers.

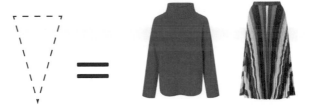

If it's the other way around, and you're a triangle, then flourish via a jacket, blouse, or sweater.

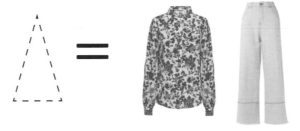

If you are pretty much in proportion then take your pick; flourish as you see fit.

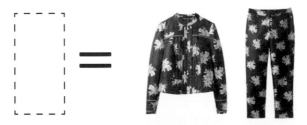

approved full-length mirror of yours to look—really look—at yourself in particular colors, patterns, and styles. Examine yourself afresh, but also with foreknowledge. Gradually you will become better at evaluating what works for you and what doesn't.

There's hair to factor in, too. Of course it becomes trickier if your hair color is not your natural one. A good hair colorist will make it their mission to render you a version of blonde or brunette that chimes as much as possible with your skin tone. But there are, alas, a fair few bad hair colorists out there. So too many of us spend years with hair that works against our complexion rather than flatters it.

Bad enough in itself, even without considering the domino effect when it comes to wearing colorful clothes. Because how do you determine "your" colors if your dyed hair already isn't one of them? If you suspect this might be the case then you need to shop around for a new hair colorist, too. Get it right and your hair will be the ultimate built-in flourish: far more useful than even the most fabulous of hussar-style jackets.

160

TRICKS OF THE TRADE

Some specifics on the nature of that attention-grabbing: Power pieces wave a flag not only generally, but also in a focused way, leading the eye to the section of the body that has been thus garbed; making that section look more than the sum of its parts. This means that, used wisely, they are doubly our friends, giving us the means to endow our figure with a proportionality it perhaps does not naturally enjoy.

If your top half is larger than your lower—if you are an inverted triangle, or a variation on the theme thereof—focus the flourishing on skirts and trousers. If it's the other way round, and you're a triangle, then flourish via a jacket, blouse, or sweater. If you are pretty much in proportion—curse you!—then take your pick; flourish as you see fit.

Bear in mind, too, the subterfuge potential of stripes. A vertically striped power piece will make that part of the body look

use proportion of your body

longer and slimmer. Lateral stripes can deliver curves where there aren't any. Diagonal stripes—one of fashion's stealth miracle workers—can cover up all sorts of lumps and bumps.

SIGNATURE STYLE
Bracelets Nails Rings

Once you have ascertained which bit of you should be iced like a cake, then you need to decide how best to do it. If your frame shape—different from your frame size—is angular, then your power pieces should be, too. A tailored jacket on top. Or sharply cut pants down below. If you are rounded then you want more draping lines and fabrics. If you are interjacent then, again, lucky you—you can veer either way. (See p.30.)

It may be that you go more particular yet, and identify a signature piece, a way in which you will flourish over and again. So not just a tailored jacket but, say, a tuxedo style, which you buy in different colors and/or trims. Or a softer, more casual utility style, the olive amped-up with assorted forms of embellishment, here embroidery, there beading.

Or not just a statement skirt, but a pleated one, in a hot hue, a metallic, or a pattern. Or you could make silk trousers your thing, in an array of different colors and prints. Delicious. For the warmer months you might have fun with traditionally winter patterns over light fabrics. Animal print or houndstooth over silk or cotton separates—be it on your top half or your bottom—looks effortlessly now. However special the piece, wear it easily, breezily, and regularly. That's how to make it your own and to get your money's worth.

And make sure that you always buy your power piece with a view to the other clothes you have in your wardrobe with which it will work. That is the point of the genre: that it augments and ornaments what you already have; more than this, that it augments and ornaments you.

Handbags / Shoes / Scarves / Jopper Coats / Jewelery Hair accessories

161

162

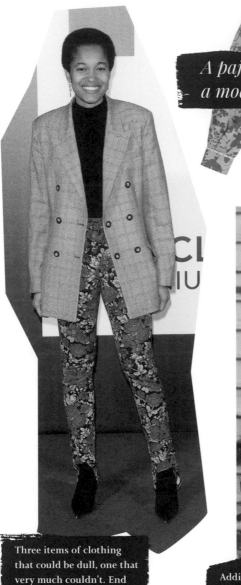

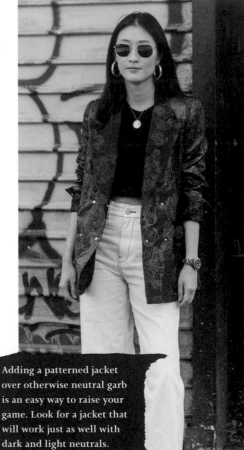

A pajama-style top is a modern classic

Three items of clothing that could be dull, one that very much couldn't. End result, dynamite.

Adding a patterned jacket over otherwise neutral garb is an easy way to raise your game. Look for a jacket that will work just as well with dark and light neutrals.

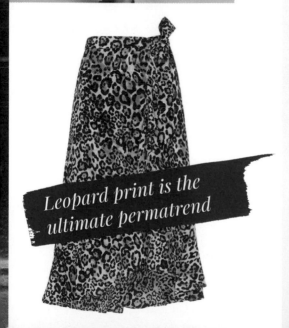

Utility wear with tweaks—like this amped-up utility jacket—is perfect for a flourish that still appears relaxed.

REASONS TO BE CHEERFUL

That's what the passion pieces in your wardrobe should be. Things that make you happy just to look at in your closet, never mind actually to wear. Identify the colors and types of patterns that you love, and that love you. Think about which part(s) of your body you like to emphasize. Consider developing a signature piece, a particular item that you buy in several colors. Then head out for some flourish shopping.

What's great about the flourish approach is it never appears try-hard. If one item is look-at-me, everything else can be more low-key.

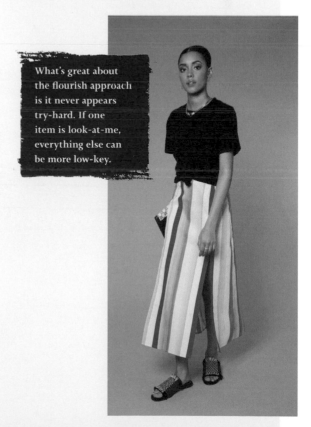

Leopard print is the ultimate permatrend

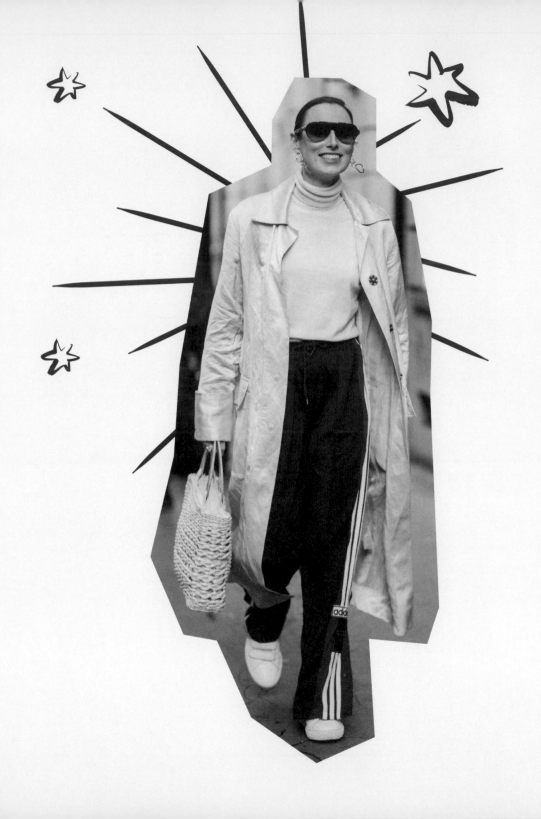

Athleisure

THE GOOD, THE BAD, AND THE UGLY

Athleisure. What a nasty hybrid of a word. And, for many, what a nasty hybrid of a concept. Certainly that's what I used to think. Sports clothing was best saved for—surprise, surprise—sports. For running in the park or downward-dogging at the yoga studio. And not for anything or anywhere else.

Bumbling around in a tracksuit away from the athletics track was for the slobs of this world, and therefore absolutely not for me. Even when I am relaxing, even when I am going no further than my sofa, I want my clothes to make me feel better about myself, not worse.

But I have completely changed my mind about athleisure in recent years. Because, yes, athleisure has been around for years now. And it is going nowhere. It's a true permatrend. The designer Tommy Hilfiger, one of the originators of the genre, talks of the "casualization" of the world, and athleisure—along with denim—has played a part in that. "In the beginning it was just about being relaxed," he told me recently. "Now it's also about being cool. People want to look like they're going to the gym even if they aren't! If you don't look at least a bit sporty, you can seem out of touch."

That's why in both Los Angeles and Silicon Valley—the two most potent spheres of visual influence of our age—it's rare to meet someone who isn't channeling at least an edge of athleisure. As Hilfiger observed, "In Silicon Valley you won't find a jacket or a tie, a blouse or a skirt. Casual has become a way of dressing for real life." And in the more forward-looking workplaces it's become a new variety of power dressing. Why? Because it's genius at delivering a youthful edge, a frisson of cool, in this era in which we are obsessed with both.

It's about more than that. Fewer and fewer of us are prepared to wear clothes that inhibit our lives. The origin of sportswear was, of course, to make it easier to move, to breathe. Yet, until remarkably recently, fashion—particularly women's fashion—tended to get in the way of just that; of living life to the fullest. As we all know, nipped-waists and tight skirts (or indeed very full

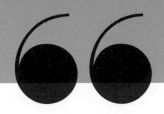

People want to look like they're going to the gym even if they aren't! If you don't look at least a bit sporty, you can seem out of touch.

—TOMMY HILFIGER

On logos

Logos are having a moment. But to my mind it is precisely that: not for the long-haul. Certainly, it's not a look for me. And I would suggest that if you are no longer in your teens it is not a look for you either. Why wear what is in essence someone else's name? You are you.

Thankfully there is at least as much athleisure out there without logos. What's more, this tends to be the stuff that's been properly revisited, tweaked to look and feel both upscale and adult, and to work with a woman's curves.

What I do have time for is the more sophisticated variety of slogan sweatshirt or tee—something else that is having a moment, a moment that has been going on for so long now that it may well prove to be another permatrend.

The trick is to choose the classiest top you can find—in terms of cut, fabric, and color—and the smartest slogan. No pictures. There are some wonderful examples out there, with words ranging from witty to wise, quirky to inspiring.

If a particular slogan really speaks to you—makes you laugh, think, or a bit of both—wear it! It's an expression of you, not a brand. And that, to my mind, is what fashion is all about.

ones), don't make the day-to-day easy. Until the 1960s a "respectable" woman couldn't even wear pants, and then it could still make waves (see p.184).

So-called "streetwear" was the first reinvention of sportswear, worn by musicians and others in the 1980s. Here was a way to look cool and feel comfortable. But it was wholesale appropriation of the original garb; no clever retool for those of us who work in an office rather than as a hip-hop artist.

SEVEN-DAY-A-WEEK PERFORMANCE WEAR

Yes, we had to wait a while before these types of clothing were adequately retooled to transcend pure functionality and become flattering, too. The fact that this has finally happened is why I have come around. Because, in short, athleisure has come around. The best of it has fully developed the leisure dimension originally promised but not quite delivered by the nomenclature, and in so doing become properly grown up, properly appropriate for the real world, not only the gym.

169

Now athleisure can be bought in thin fabrics that drape softly rather than adding bulk. And some of its wonderfully practical detailing has been redesigned to look fantastic, too. Now I can find athleisure that makes me appear cool and *sportif*, but also just as sleek and chic as if I were wearing a suit.

Take the much-maligned elasticized waist, for example. Nothing comfier and, of yore, nothing less becoming. These days it is possible to find an elasticized waist that you can bespoke in a way that suits you best, perhaps flattening it out over the stomach and/or your bottom, but still benefiting from that user-friendly ruching elsewhere.

Yes, the canniest designers are now producing athleisure that is designed to enhance the female figure. They are actually tailoring pieces that were originally the very the opposite of tailored. Tailored athleisure. Sounds mad, but it is one of the most sensible things to have happened in fashion in years. And certainly one of the most happy-making.

Clothes that feel comfortable and relaxed, but that also make you look your best. Clothes that effortlessly modernize your wardrobe, not to mention shave years off your birth certificate, should you be of an age or inclination to consider that a good thing. What's not to like?

THE HEAVEN'S IN THE DETAIL

But it's all in the execution. More specifically, it's all about those fabrics. When it comes to the top half, anyone with a bust needs to avoid a conventional sweatshirt, and everyone needs to balance it out with a sleek lower half. For me, the cannier route it to buy a sweatshirt-styled thin sweater, or even a silk sweatshirt or tee. A thin zip-up funnel-neck top—jersey or wool—worn under a jacket, or even under a dress, is another route. A thin hoodie—yes, hoodie—layered under tailoring is one more. And, oh yes, did I mention that all of the above should be thin?

Or how about a luxe bomber jacket? The atelier of the London-based couturier Anna Valentine is a symphony of stealth chic, filled with beauteous chiffon dresses and immaculately cut tailoring. It also majors heavily on bomber jackets, which have been reinvented courtesy of princess-worthy fabrics and embellishment. "It's a solution to what to put around your shoulders in the evening that isn't the dreaded bolero. It's a more modern take," says Valentine.

When it comes to the bottom half, the same rules apply. Thin cotton jersey track pants get a tick from me, chunky cotton jersey ones don't. My biggest tick is for satin or crepe iterations, perhaps with some definitively nonathleisure detailing,

Worried that you are too old for all of the above? You are not. It's all about what you wear them with. Because the other key to making athleisure work for you is to mix it with contrasting pieces. Satin track pants plus tailored jacket and an elegant mid-heel is a youth-endowing take on the pantsuit, and great for the office. Satin track pants plus crisp white shirt, higher heels, and chandelier earrings will render you the coolest woman at any cocktail party at which you might find yourself. Truly.

Absolutely yes

It might sound like a contradiction in terms, chic athleisure. But it's one of the easiest ways to look both pulled together and youthful. Make sure your athleisure is suitably upscale, and add some streamlined tailoring.

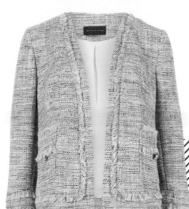

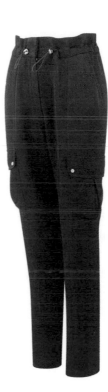

TAILORED JACKET

SATIN TRACK
PANTS

HEELS

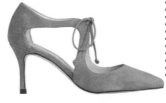

ATHLUXE: THE GLAM APPROACH

These days you can find gorgeously upscale iterations of athleisure. The Italian label Dolce & Gabbana, for example, reliably sends a dozen or so takes on the track pant down its catwalk every season. "If you look at the new generation, they don't wear denim," Stefano Gabbana told me recently. "The new denim is the track pant."

How does the label endow them with the kind of glamour a Dolce & Gabbana customer expects? By delivering them in lace, or studding them with diamanté, or embroidering them to within an inch of their fabulous lives. More affordable versions of all the above are available on a high street near you.

Embellishment has become a primary way to elevate the kind of practical clothing that most of us demand. That's why athleisure can be found with almost every square inch adorned, as can denim, shirting, and utility wear. I love embellishment, but the key is always to wear one blinged-out piece, and then keep everything else simple. I have a pair of navy wool crepe track pants trimmed with sequins that I wear with a plain navy crew neck or a white blouse, or maybe both; nothing more. I finish off the look with either sneakers or heels, depending on my mood and/or my calendar.

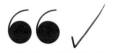

The key is always to wear one blinged-out piece, and then keep everything else simple.

Still not sure athleisure is for you? A bit of sporty detailing is all you need to benefit from athleisure voodoo. (Yes, its effects really are that magical.) A zipper here, a ribbed neckline there. The ultimate one-stop way to change up an otherwise nonathleisure ensemble is a great pair of sneakers. Wear them with bare legs and transform everything from a floral dress to a pantsuit into, age-depending, cool-girl or cool-woman.

INTRODUCING THE ATHDRESS

I am hoping the resisters might be coming around to the idea of athleisure by this stage. But if you are someone who doesn't wear pants, you may still be thinking it is not for you. *Au contraire.* There are some beautiful jersey dresses now available, some with a drawstring waist, some just waiting to be belted or allowed to flow free.

Or you can go dressier, picking up a more tailored dress with subtle athleisure detailing in the form of a zipped collar. If you are still not confident about pulling off upscale athleisure, still worried it is not feminine enough, or that it will look too dressed-down for your purposes, buying one head-to-toe piece that will do all the genre-busting for you is a great way to change things up. Wear with pretty flats or mid-heels for that scary Monday morning meeting, with white sneakers for that jolly Sunday dinner with friends.

If you are still not confident about pulling off upscale athleisure, buying one head-to-toe piece that will do all the genre-busting for you is a great way to change things up.

A frock isn't the only route for you pant-eschewers. As you gain confidence, don't forget about the mix-and-non-match approach (see Chapter 7), in the form of a chic, sleek skirt given a fresh edge by way of a tee or sweatshirt, or sweatshirt-styled sweater. I threw a birthday brunch when I last hit 21—amazing how it keeps on coming around—and wore a white cotton slogan tee with a tasselled black pencil skirt that wouldn't look out of place at the Moulin Rouge. I could have worn white sneakers, too, but instead matched my style of accessories to the skirt rather than the top: black lace flats, and dramatic multi-pearl drop earrings. What was the slogan on that tee? "Stéréotype." That it was written in French added a certain, ahem, *je ne sais quoi,* I like to think. But, more importantly, the

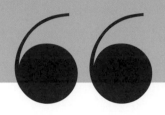

If you look at the new generation, they don't wear denim. The new denim is the track pant.

—STEFANO GABBANA

irony of that statement was clear. Dressed with such a disregard for what were once the sartorial rules of engagement, I looked anything but stereotypical.

But did I look good? My late grandmothers would have reeled in bafflement, I imagine. But I received a definitive thumbs-up from all in attendance that day, male and female, and my close friends—most of whom do not work in fashion—are not the sort to pull their punches when it comes to what I wear. (Or anything else for that matter!) Indeed a number of women told me they would never have thought of such unlikely outfit-fellows, but were going to give a similar ensemble a test-wear as a result. The reports back have been highly favorable. I rest my case.

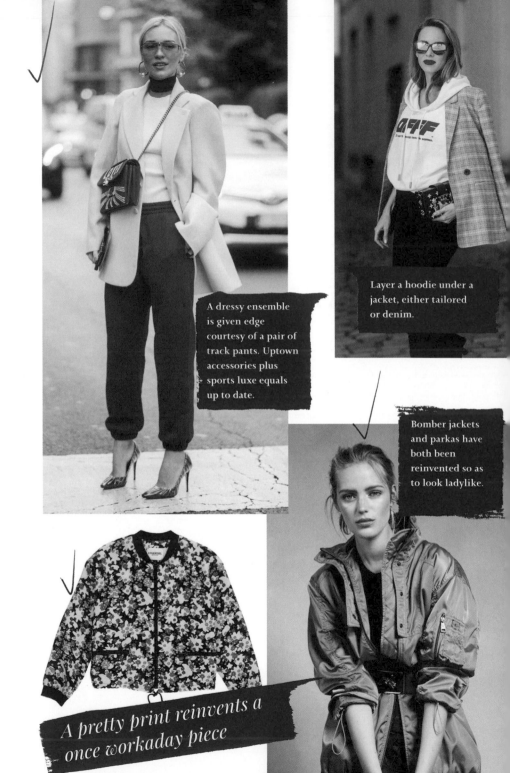

A dressy ensemble is given edge courtesy of a pair of track pants. Uptown accessories plus sports luxe equals up to date.

Layer a hoodie under a jacket, either tailored or denim.

Bomber jackets and parkas have both been reinvented so as to look ladylike.

A pretty print reinvents a once workaday piece

PLAY THE GAME

Where to start with athleisure? With just one piece per outfit. That's more than enough to benefit from the genre's freshness. But how to make sure you look chic as well as cool? By always counterbalancing with another item that's super-polished, like a gorgeous handbag or heels. Or by ensuring that your chosen item of athleisure can deliver said polish all by itself. Think silk and satin, feminine pattern, and embellishment.

Box-fresh is the way to go

Pairing sports luxe with something more feminine like this pleated skirt is softening.

Track pants in a thin, flattering fabric have become among the most useful items in my wardrobe. Easy to dress up or down.

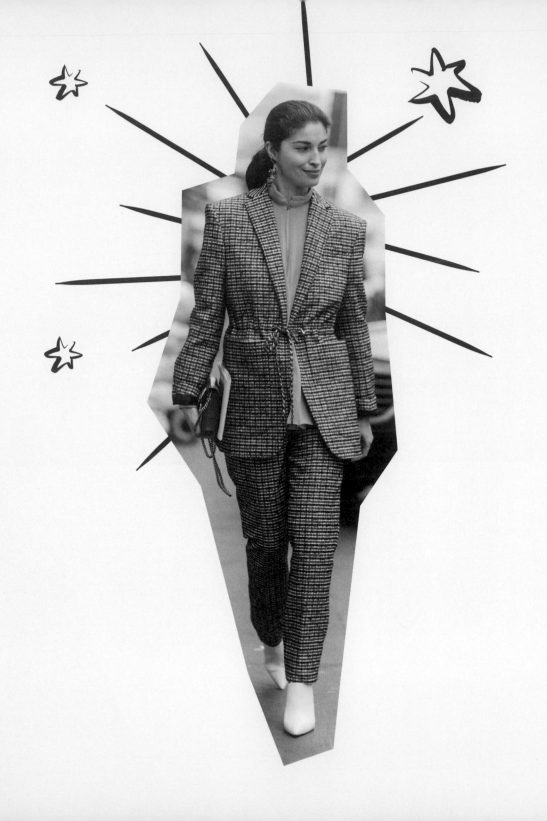

12

Working
It

HOW TO DRESS WITH MONDAY-TO-FRIDAY CONFIDENCE

Dress to impress. Sounds an old-fashioned idea. Yet it's anything but, especially when it comes to working life.

Clothes matter in the workplace because people draw conclusions from them, often without even being aware that they are doing so. You just need to make sure that the conclusions they are reaching courtesy of your wardrobe are the right ones.

It's also worth noting that the kind of conclusions they are led to by a particular outfit today might be very different from only a decade ago. In the 21st century, blending in too much—looking overly conformist—can damage you more than standing out. Most modern companies don't want yes men and women, and your clothes can mark you as an independent thinker, as someone worth listening to, and—before you know it—promoting.

As Virginia Woolf wrote in her novel *Orlando* in 1928, "Vain trifles as they seem, clothes have, they say, more important offices than merely to keep us warm. They change our view of the world and the world's view of us." This is why what you wear to work should be more than just an office-appropriate uniform. It should be part of your arsenal. "Dress like you are going to meet your worst enemy today," is how Coco Chanel once put it. And that wasn't even for the office. Imagine her on the topic of Monday-to-Friday garb. Terrifying.

FIRST IMPRESSIONS

In his best-selling book *Blink: The Power of Thinking Without Thinking*, Malcolm Gladwell looks at the high-speed subconscious processing we humans use, much of which is based on visual clues. It can take us seconds to make up our mind about a new person, and once we have done so, well, we have done so. A mind made up is precisely that. It may be right, it may be wrong, but it's inescapable: how you look, how you dress, matters.

In most workplaces a process of evaluation is ongoing. Which can feel stressful looked at in one light, but in another offers exciting opportunities for advancement. It's never too late, in other words, or at least it shouldn't be, and if you suspect it might be, it's time to move on.

"

Vain trifles as they seem, clothes have, they say, more important offices than merely to keep us warm. They change our view of the world and the world's view of us.

— *ORLANDO, VIRGINIA WOOLF*

Sure, the intricacies of your attire may vary depending on where you work. Every office has its own codes, and first off it behooves you to work out what they are. Indeed, one of the most useful skills you can develop en route to finding your style more generally is to look closely at other people. Observe your colleagues as an anthropologist might, because they are—whether aware of it or not—a kind of tribe. There may well be outliers, people who deliberately stand out through their clothing choices, but there will be a middle ground. Plot it carefully. Do the women wear pants or dresses and skirts? If the latter, what is the default skirt length? What about heel heights? Is the overall look polished or more laid back? What chimes with your personal style and what doesn't?

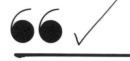

You want to blend in and stand out at one and the same time. Sounds impossible, but it can be done.

How can you dress to fit in, but also—just as importantly—to stand out? Because among your colleagues there will be one or two women at least who have got a style signature which is their office equivalent of that hi-vis jacket again (see pp.60–61). And hi-vis dressing is important for the woman on the way up. You want to figure out what your version is. You want to blend in and stand out at one and the same time. Sounds impossible, but it can be done.

Your hi-vis jacket might, in fact, be just that, by which I don't mean the bright orange affair favored by road sweepers, but a similarly hot-hued blazer, sharply tailored in wool, with defined shoulders to make you feel strong. Those padded shoulders ape the top-heavy triangularity of a muscular body; they signal physical strength. The shape-shifting abilities of the power jacket makes it my favorite office miracle worker.

American designer Norma Kamali was one of the first to tweak men's tailoring for women in the 1980s. "Everyone talks about the 1970s as being the birth of feminism," she said once, "but for me the '80s were really about feminism in practical use. The silhouette I was doing—broad shoulders and thin hips—was my way of reinterpreting masculine power, but with humor."

Our subconscious—and that of the people we work with—registers that semaphoring, even if we don't realize it's happening. We feel different in a hi-vis jacket. Colleagues look at us differently. Or it might be a hi-vis blouse, jewel-hued and worn under otherwise restrained suiting. Or a hi-vis necklace. Even a lipstick. You get the idea.

Certainly it makes sense to focus your attention on your top half because that, if you think about it, is where other people's attention tends to be focused in the office. What is seen from desk level up is what really matters. I always wear some jewelry, and/or have an interesting neckline, and/or wear some bright color, even if it's only in the form of that lipstick.

Of course, workplace attire should communicate competency, not craziness, so we are looking at flourishes, not full-on fandango, and the overall effect should be pared back and pulled together.

183

But it should absolutely not add up to boring. That is the most common mistake people make when dressing for the office. You don't want to blend into the background. You want to stand out. You don't want to look anonymous. You want to look like you at your most dynamic.

> # What is seen from desk level up is what really matters.

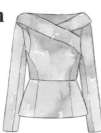

SEIZING OUR DAY

You also want to look like a woman, not like a version of a man. We live, lucky us, in an era when the particularities of what women have to offer the world—be it a softer, more empathetic form of power, or a variety of networking based on genuine communality as well as healthy competition—is finally being recognized and sought out.

Don't render your womanliness invisible. Celebrate it. Let the men dress boringly if they must. But don't ape them in their dreary entirety. Wear a black or gray pantsuit if you want to, but change it up with outsize pearl earrings, with mascaraed eyelashes, some embellished flats, or even—office depending—sneakers, provided they are squeaky clean.

That said, never look *too* womanly, in the sense of revealing too much flesh. A skirt that is too short or a *décolletage* that is too low will make you stand out for the wrong reasons. As designer Diane von Furstenberg once observed to me, "When you work you want to look good, you want to look strong. You want to show off your body—why not? But not in a way that will make men objectify you." And relish how far we have come. Trailblazing 1960s fashion editor Felicity Green, the first woman on the board of a British newspaper, now in her 90s, told me there was a furore when she first wore trousers in the *Daily Mirror* offices. A male colleague of hers later recalled that, "All female staff were expected to wear skirts or dresses. Felicity turned up one day in a trouser suit. The editor was shocked but the dam had broken and the girls [sic] began following Felicity's example."

Green had more freedom than the other women at the company, most of whom were secretaries. But even she conceded to me that, "When I wore a skirt I had a much easier time." That's not, alas, an impossible conclusion for some of us to draw even now. But the situation—trouser-related and beyond—has improved immeasurably.

GETTING IT RIGHT

What ticks the contemporary box perfectly? A colorful pantsuit is on point, perhaps softened with a silk pussy-bow blouse. Suiting makes you look like serious stuff, and rendered in a colorful fabric it also makes you

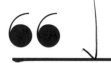

Suiting makes you look like serious stuff, and rendered in a colorful fabric it also makes you look interesting.

Nice and smartly does it

♡ *Squeaky clean is generally the only way to go.*
♡ *Never wear anything that looks scruffy or shabby.*
♡ *Never wear a black that's turned yellow, or a white that's turned gray.*
♡ *When in doubt, refresh.*
♡ *You don't want to come across as outmoded, so it's important that your clothes don't either.*
♡ *Chanel again: "Dress shabbily and they remember the dress; dress impeccably and they remember the woman."*

BORING!!!

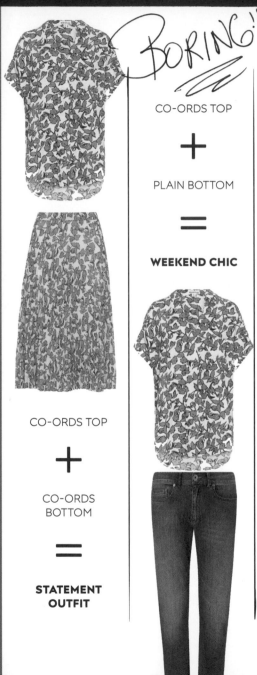

CO-ORDS TOP

+

PLAIN BOTTOM

=

WEEKEND CHIC

CO-ORDS TOP

+

CO-ORDS BOTTOM

=

STATEMENT OUTFIT

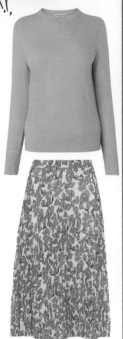

PLAIN TOP

+

CO-ORDS BOTTOM

=

OFFICE ELEGANT

Items that will mix and match you through the week are the canniest purchases around. That's what makes co-ords so great.

look interesting. Plus colorful doesn't have to mean bright. A forest green or petrol blue is enough of a statement of difference.

"Co-ords" (see p.107) are another way to look effortlessly pulled together. Co-ords tend to be patterned rather than plain, so are great for making a bold statement. They also offer extra flexibility, as you can wear them separately with a contrast half. Co-ords on your top half plus jeans for example. Great for the weekend. Co-ords on your bottom half plus cashmere crewneck. Great for any time, work or play.

A jumpsuit is another indubitably 21st-century way to pull off office chic. It works like a suit, but looks up to date, and contrasts with the boys. Keep color and pattern dialed back here. Indeed, the savviest way to play the office jumpsuit game is to pick one in a classic fabric that gives a sly nod to what used to be strictly men-only—a navy and white pinstripe perhaps, or gray wool.

When it comes to a dress many women feel a tailored sheath style is the only way to go, especially in more male-dominated, suit-led environments, such as the law and the finance. The sheath is a suit in dress's clothing. But if you are not careful it can look dated. Search out modernizing add-ons like an athleisure zipper or two; contrast seaming; some kind of detail at the waist, perhaps a band of fabric, perhaps a matching tie belt or contrast ribbon. For certain body shapes the sheath is also not as flattering as we've been led to think. If you are pear-shaped, for example, it can draw attention to your hips. Better to pick a full skirt and a nipped-in waist. Or to overlay a jacket that gives balancing emphasis to your shoulders.

187

CREATIVE CLOTHES

Have you considered the so-called power floral? This is a reinvention of the once-girlish tea-dress, which has more recently become a favorite in the creative industries. It's revealing of the semantics of dress still in play that many of us subconsciously eschew such feminine dressing in the workplace. Where are the women politicians wearing florals, for example? For the moment, absolutely nowhere.

But if you pick a print that's strong rather than pallid (a power floral typically comes with a dark or bright background), if you accessorize with footwear that is the opposite of spindly (perhaps—spot the theme—some power boots), if you sling over a blazer (that power jacket again), and add on a cross-body bag, you will look like you are going places professionally, whatever your work milieu. As a result—assuming you have the small matter of the job itself in hand, of course—like as not, you soon will be.

Indeed, there is much to be learned from the denizens of advertising agencies, the film industry, magazines, and the like. You may not want to go full-on *Ugly Betty*, but you can pick up some ideas, and tweak accordingly. So here's my report from the creative frontlines. These are women who embrace all of the looks already discussed. They also add into the mix upscale athleisure, in the form of silky track pants and thin hoodies and sweatshirts (see Chapter 11). And they love the easy-breezy appeal of a neat sweater with a skirt—perhaps a pencil, perhaps a long, pleated or floaty asymmetric style. Then they overlay a blazer, sleeved or sleeveless, or a vest, or a bomber. And they play with contrasting textures. That sweater might be mohair; that skirt, silk; that blazer enriched with some embroidered detailing.

What's more, if they aren't a column, a rectangle, or a rounded body shape, these women often have something akin to a belt wardrobe, half a dozen or so different options at least. They know a belt is a great way to change up any outfit and deliver a professional edge. Imagine a long, thin cardigan over a pencil skirt and pussy-bow blouse, perhaps with some pretty all-day-long kitten heels. Add a thick wasp-waist-endowing belt, perhaps in black leather, perhaps black elastic with on-trend utility buckle. Immediately you look corner-office-appropriate. Swap out the pencil skirt for chic track pants. Keep everything else the same. Ditto, but with added modernity. Think back to that aforementioned power-floral dress. Add belt. It looks more powerful again.

Women in the creative industries walk the line between the dressy and the casual, and it is this that makes them look modern,

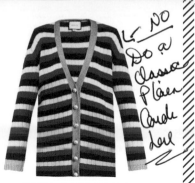

NO
Do a
Classic
Plain
Cardi
Luv

THIN CARDIGAN

+

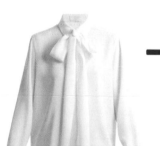

BLOUSE

+

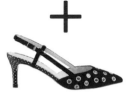

KITTEN HEELS

When shopping for separates buy pieces you can dial up or down for maximum flexibility.

+

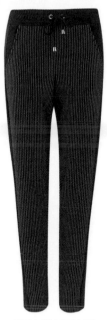

TRACK PANT

OR

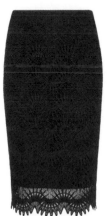

PENCIL SKIRT

go-getting, like the kind of person who should be in charge, if they aren't already. But, importantly, the end result is always—always—more elegant than casual. Because this is what really ensures they look like boss class.

How do they pull it off? By only wearing clothes in perfect condition, and in the best—for which read "softest"—fabrics they can afford. By investing in top-notch accessories, be it shoes or bags, and looking after them. And, again, by changing them up the second they are past their best. By dressing interestingly, originally, but looking the opposite of try-hard. It needs to appear effortless. Because that is what will help your rise appear effortless. Yes, strange as it may seem, looking like you can deliver will make you believe you can do just that, and that will make other people believe you can. And then you will. *for sure!*

THE FASHION POWER POSE

Dressing the part has a similar effect to the so-called "power pose" social psychologist Amy Cuddy talked about in her much-watched Ted Talk in 2012. Standing in a wide stance with your hands on your hips in best Wonder Woman style—yes, her again—is one example.

Since then some have dismissed Cuddy's research as pseudo-science, but she is standing firm; posing powerfully, in fact. "Dozens of researchers at universities around the world have conducted experiments looking at the effects of adopting expansive postures on emotional, cognitive, behavioral, and physiological outcomes," she said in a follow-up interview in 2017. "What's absolutely clear from the studies is that adopting expansive poses increases people's feelings of power and confidence. And feeling powerful is a critical psychological variable." And feeling powerful produces a range of consequences, continues Cuddy, "including improved executive functioning, optimism, creativity, authenticity, the ability to self-regulate, and performance in various domains, to name a handful."

Clothes can do that for you, too. Bring on the fashion power pose.

Game-changer dressing

The charity Smart Works offers a great example of what happens when someone looks, literally, the business. It helps women who have struggled to find a job for years, women who are referred to the charity via other charities, job centers, prisons, and the National Health Service. "The one thing these women have in common," says co-founder Juliet Hughes-Hallett, "is that they have no confidence. When they go for a job for which they have the right qualifications, and they still don't get it, that is why."

Hughes-Hallett and her team of volunteers ask each woman how she wants to look for her interview, and then, courtesy of racks of donated clothes, try to deliver it as closely as possible. "When they stand in front of the mirror in their new outfit it's a real hair-standing-on-end moment. You can see them thinking, 'My God, this might actually be possible'. It is like they have put on a suit of armor."

Next the women receive coaching on how to succeed at an interview. But it's that mirror reveal which is, says Hughes-Hallett, the real game-changer point. "It is the ultimate illustration of what clothes can do for the self-esteem." Sixty percent of the women who come to Smart Works get a job shortly afterward.

192

Choose a suit that's anything but predictable, and you can enjoy the best of both worlds.

Power boots

A black blazer appears freshly womanly courtesy of a tie-waist.

Looking both chic and relaxed can get you a long way. A cross-body bag is hard to beat. So are leg-lengthening side-stripe trousers.

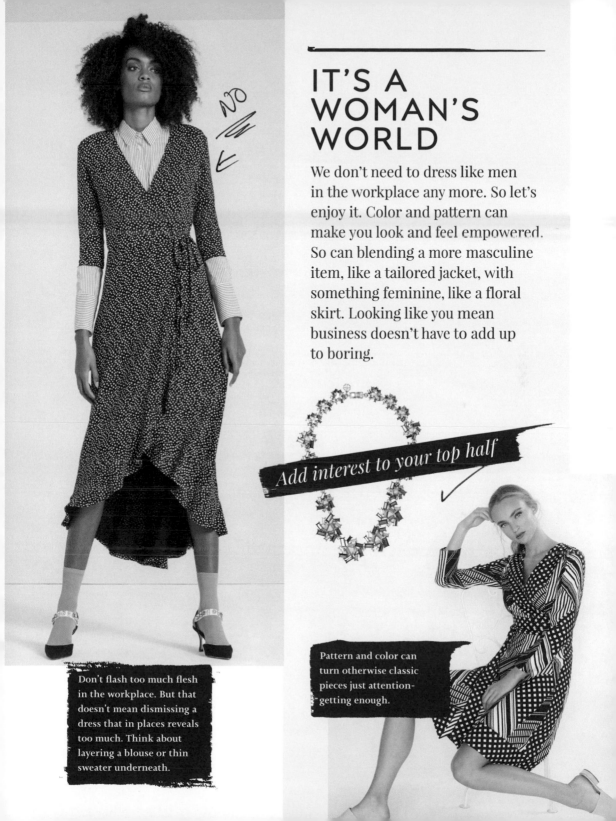

IT'S A WOMAN'S WORLD

We don't need to dress like men in the workplace any more. So let's enjoy it. Color and pattern can make you look and feel empowered. So can blending a more masculine item, like a tailored jacket, with something feminine, like a floral skirt. Looking like you mean business doesn't have to add up to boring.

Add interest to your top half

Don't flash too much flesh in the workplace. But that doesn't mean dismissing a dress that in places reveals too much. Think about layering a blouse or thin sweater underneath.

Pattern and color can turn otherwise classic pieces just attention-getting enough.

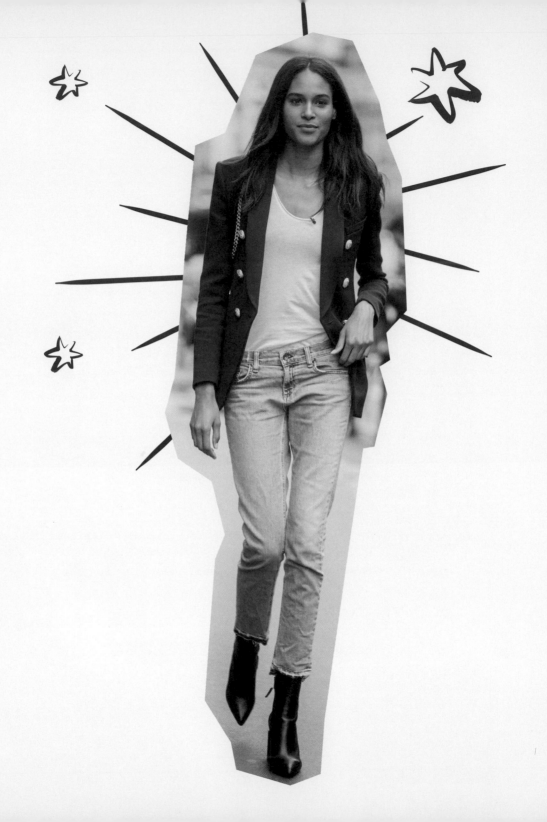

13

The Right *Pants,* The Perfect *Jeans*

YES, THEY'RE OUT THERE, AND HERE'S HOW TO FIND THEM

They are the great divider, not just literally but metaphorically. I meet many women who love pants and/or jeans, and live in them. I meet just as many who loathe them, and avoid them, particularly women who are larger, who don't like their hips, bottoms, and/or thighs.

The vast majority of the fashion pack are pant-lovers. "Now I always wear trousers," says Emmanuelle Alt, the editor of French *Vogue*. "They are just so easy." Of course they are easy for the willowy Alt. Pant-shopping for skinny-minnies is a walk in the park, comparatively speaking. For the rest of us it's work in the park, if not a full-on workout. But once you have found pants that flatter you and that are comfortable, then you, too, can enjoy the ease they deliver.

THE HERSTORY

It's worth noting what a recent phenomenon pants for women in the West are, and how for a long time most of us weren't allowed to wear strides, freedom-giving clothes that, as this synonym suggests, enable you to stride; to go places.

In Eastern countries women have worn them under tunics for centuries. But in Britain the pant-wearing so-called "pit-brow lasses" working above-ground in the coalfields of 19th-century industrial Lancashire were such a novelty that local photographic studios sold postcards of them to visitors.

Around the same time in America a campaign was begun to liberate women from their restrictive clothing via the adoption of Turkish-style pantaloons. One early advocate was Amelia Bloomer, owner of the *The Lily*, the first newspaper by and for women. Bloomer encouraged this way of dressing for her readers, hence the pants became known as "bloomers." This led to the so-called Bloomer Craze of 1851, complete with bloomer parties, bloomer festivals, and—wait for it—bloomer institutes. In Britain the cause was taken up by the Rational Dress Movement.

But it took nearly a century before pants were worn in great numbers, when many women worked outside the home for the first time during World War II. Even then *Vogue* insisted that pant-wearers must be under 50 and under 140 pounds, and it was—unbelievably—an ongoing subject of national debate in the newspapers whether "slacks" would turn British women slack.

Two decades after that the trailblazing fashion editor Felicity Green was met with amazement when she wore pants to the *Daily Mirror* offices. It was this, among other things, that inspired her most celebrated front page, in which she outlined to the paper's 5 million readers why 1964 was "The year that changed our lives." "Khrushchev sacked, China explodes atomic bomb …" was the opening large-font gambit. And then, 10 lines of serious geopolitics later … "And of course, skirts got shorter, boys' hair got longer, smart girls wore the trousers, the topless went bust and the Beatles (who else?) went everywhere …"

Yes, women wearing pants used to make the front page. And it's not as if the issue has entirely been laid to rest even now. Some schools still insist that their female pupils wear skirts or dresses. But, in general, these days we can wear the pants, should we so choose. So why do some of us choose not to? Mainly because it can be a struggle to find a fit that flatters you. But, trust me, it can be done, and it is worth doing.

The solution is to buy to fit the biggest part and then alter the rest.

YOU ARE NEVER TOO BIG FOR A GREAT PAIR OF PANTS

Many of us on the front row—myself included—have, to quote an American peer of mine, "plenty in the trunk." So how do we find pants that work with our boot(y)? The most common problem is that a pair that fits around the thighs doesn't fit at the waist, or vice versa. That's certainly always been my issue.

The solution is to buy to fit the biggest part and then alter the rest. It's that simple. That's what the fashion crowd do across the board with their clothes. It costs more money, of course, but it's one of the most significant changes you can make in terms of finding your way to, to paraphrase Milan Kundera, an eternal lightness of dressing.

If you are very slim you may need to get extra fabric—or *wings*—taken in from the outsides of the hips, or any excess around the inner thighs or crotch. You don't want to look droopy or waif-like.

Don't see getting things altered as an admission of defeat. It's impossible for even the best-intentioned brand to create sizes that work for everyone. You only need to look around the changing room at the swimming pool to see the myriad variations on the theme of a size 12, and any other size you could care to mention. And then there is the issue of vanity sizing. Some brands are in the business of making their customers feel smaller by putting a smaller number on a big size. I know a sylph of a stylist who insists she can be four different sizes, depending on what brand she is trying. My issue tends to be that I sit between two sizes, so now—as discussed—I buy bigger and adapt accordingly.

DON'T FORGET THE REST

Remember, too, that you are choosing an item of clothing that doesn't only have to work on its own, but also with many of the other items in your wardrobe. People think buying separates is easier than buying, say, a dress. It's actually harder, because a pair of pants is just one piece in a bigger jigsaw, and if that piece doesn't fit, then the whole thing goes wrong.

Part of it is about aesthetics. Most brands deliver a handful of modes of dressing well. Shopping within one brand for a head-to-toe look is an easy way to ensure that the feel of the different pieces you are wearing chime together. Part of it is about proportions. Whatever your size or shape, remember that you want to skim, not swamp; that's how to bring it under control (see p.28). Very wide-leg trousers will merely draw attention to

The pants policy

When you try on an item and like it, that's
when you apply the pants policy.

First scrunch up the fabric to see if it creases.

*Then enact the 20-minute trial. That's how long
you wear them for, and during that time you
walk around, sit down, do jumping jacks. OK, I
made that last one up, but you get the idea. You
want to put your putative purchase through its
paces before it's too late.*

♡ *How do they look?*
♡ *Have they gone saggy around
the waist or bottom?*
♡ *Is the fabric exhibiting any signs of
wear and tear?*
♡ *Has even a smidgen of the dread camel toe
made an appearance?*
♡ *Has the leg length stayed the same as initially,
or has it gone shorter or longer?*

your thigh width; better by far to wear a less wide or a straight leg. If you have a waist, emphasize it. "Bringing everything in at the waist is flattering," says the red-carpet stylist Rebecca Corbin-Murray. "For me it's all about rediscovering the waist."

THE NITTY-GRITTY

You tend to get what you pay for when it comes to pants. Or rather, good pants are rarely cheap, but bad pants can often be expensive. Look for fabrics with some stretch, whatever your size, and whatever the nature of your lines. Just make sure that if you are angular, the stretch fabric you choose presents as sharp rather than soft.

If possible shop in-store rather than online so that you can compare different styles and cuts, and be brutal about dismissing what doesn't work for you. Personal stylists always—and I mean always—shop in the flesh. Hit a few stores on the high street or, better still, go to a multi-brand department store. It will actually save you time in the long run. Besides, the whole point about developing your style-smarts is that you will get it right more and more often, and so need to shop less and less often as a result.

Look also for a generosity of cut, even if the style is slimline. Some of the most common problems arise from straightforward meanness in the pattern-cutting process. So-called "camel toe," for example, stems from a lack of fabric around the groin. That said, if this is a consistent problem for you, it may be that you are long in the front and/or back rise, as it's known in the trade. The rise is the measurement from the waistband to the crotch in both the front and the back. Longer than average in either of these measurements and there won't be enough fabric there for you. If you have a generously rounded bottom—that fabulous booty again—this may be impacting the length of your back rise. The designers who cut the best trousers for curvier shapes tend to offer a higher rise at the back.

THE ANKLE FLASH

Whatever the nature of your curves, bear in mind that your ankles showcase you at your slimmest. That's why the fashion pack loves cropped pants. "I always favor a trouser that hits the narrowest point of your leg between your ankle and your mid-calf," says Corbin-Murray, "and is wide, but not too wide, in the leg."

Don't make the mistake of thinking this is an approach suited only to the tall. Flashing your ankles—along with your wrists—can actually lengthen the appearance of your limbs, especially when those crops are paired with a mid-heel for extra elongation. (Just make sure—as always—that the shoe isn't clunky if you are petite.) Some decorative detailing at the hem—a trim or fringe—can also look good, but be sure to avoid roll-up versions if you are petite, or if you are tall but have short legs.

Trouser soothsayer Clare Hornby—who heads up the boutique brand Me+Em—told me she recently held a styling session for eight friends of all sizes. "Six of them ended up buying a straight-leg crop," she laughed, "even though they had all started out totally against the idea. Most women have great ankle bones, and this style really shows them off. "

The other route to making your legs appear longer is to wear your pants slightly long. The exact opposite approach in other words, but with the same end result, and useful when it comes to disguising large feet, too. Crease-front trousers will also give the appearance of length, and you can push things further still by picking shoes that are the same color. Slim cuts and higher waists will elongate as well. It's all about finessing your way to the best possible you again.

If you have heavy legs and ankles, go dark on your bottom half, and seek out straight-leg styles, slight flares, culottes, and palazzo pants, but avoid pants that are baggy or shapeless. Remember: skim not swamp. For that same reason, if you have a tummy, flat-front trousers tend to be the most flattering, provided they have enough fabric in them. (Again, buy large, then tailor.)

Front-pleat trousers aren't an absolute no-no if you are bigger. But I look for styles that are sewn down at least half way and do not balloon out if viewed from the side. A full deep pleat can make you appear larger all over. Conversely, a decorative side stripe is another miracle-working special effect when it comes to elongating the legs. The cleverest brands will even move the stripe slightly forward from where a side seam would usually lie in order to make the leg seem narrower from the front.

Be wary when it comes to side pockets—unless you have slim hips—and embrace the side zipper.

POCKETS AND THIGH GAPS

Back pockets are a whole art form. If you have a flat bottom, then large patch packets or curved pockets on the bottom will make it look rounder. (Avoid loose styles and boyfriend cuts.) If you have a large bottom then diagonal pockets, ideally long rather than short, will make it look smaller. (And wear structured styles, plus avoid clingy or stiff fabrics, and anything tight.)

> **A decorative side stripe is a miracle-working special effect when it comes to elongating the legs.**

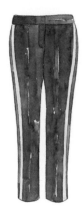

Another stealth trick of the trade is a slight tuck at the back of the pant which helps to create the illusion of a thigh gap. See how geeky you can go on this stuff? But all that really matters is that you try on the right kind of cut for your shape in the first place, and that you are prepared to buy big and alter.

As always, if pants just don't feel or look like you, then by all means ignore all of the above. Don't force yourself to join the pant-wearing classes. "Some women are just not good in trousers generally," says the personal stylist Annabel Hodin. "They look like they are in the army or a bus conductor."

yuck yuck yuck

They used to be the sensible, serious choice. Not any more. Pants come in colors and patterns galore. A flat-fronted cut with no side pockets is slimming, and cropped legs can be flattering, too. Wear with a statement shoe.

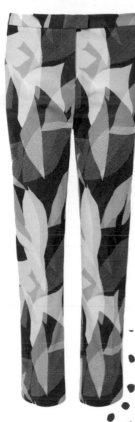

PRINT PANTS

HOT SHOES

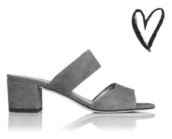

Which pockets will work for you depends on myriad infinitesimal factors. But if your bottom is big and/or flat, these are your best routes.

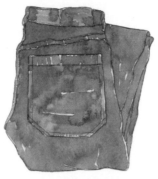

LARGE

Great for making a large derrière appear smaller, or a flat one rounder.

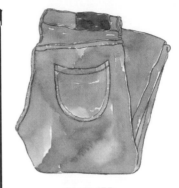

CURVED

Another way to bring added bootyliciousness to the flatter variety of booty.

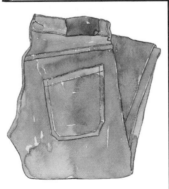

DIAGONAL

Tactic number two for dialing down the chunkier trunk. Make sure the pocket length is long, not short.

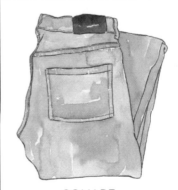

SQUARE

And diversion number three ... square pockets, again long rather than short.

JEANS GENIUS

The same goes for jeans. They have become something of a religion in our culture. If you find a pair you love and that loves you—and my plan is to help you on that one—then great. But if jeans really aren't for you, then don't sweat it. Take long-time industry professional Samantha Cameron, who now heads up her own label, Cefinn, after her former life as the Prime Minister's wife. "I love jeans on other people but they look awful on me because I've got a big bum and thighs. I just don't feel comfortable in them because they don't suit me. Instead I wear tailored trousers, or dresses."

Fashion people are good at saying no to things they really don't like; that they feel really don't suit them. It's a confidence thing. Being able to say "no" to trends—more than that in the case of denim, to fashion dogmas—is as important as being able to say "yes." You need to do it, too, be it when it comes to jeans or anything else.

The current denim domination is rather odd, if you think about it. Here is an incredibly particular—even peculiar—item of clothing originally designed for an incredibly particular purpose: namely to cope with the rough-riding, rough-living of 19th-century cowboys. Now they are ubiquitous. Why? Because they came to be seen as counter-cultural, and so were adopted in the 1950s by the new invention that was the teenager. These days, our youth-obsessed culture in which—in theory if not so much in practice—nonconformism is valued, jeans are a way of signaling our status.

But maybe you have other ways to send the message—a pair of cool shoes can do the job nicely—or a different message entirely to communicate. If so you will be in great company. When I once asked Miuccia Prada if she would ever wear jeans, she laughed in my face. She sees jeans as boring, and in a world full of diverse fabrics, with myriad colors, patterns, and textures, she may well have a point. For fellow designer Carolina Herrera it's more of an age thing. "Jeans look so good on young girls, but when you reach a certain age you have to change—no? The easiest way to look older is to dress young."

I am no fan of mutton dressed as lamb, but I think jeans can look good whatever your age. (Fashion is, by its very definition, a matter of opinion, not of diktat.) I give you, by way of gorgeous example, the 70-something Lauren Hutton. But they have to be the right jeans for you, which is the case whatever your age, be you 18 or 80.

THE MIND-BODY EQUATION

I am not going to pretend it is easy finding them. Yves Saint Laurent once said that he wished he had invented jeans, because of their "simplicity." Yeah, right. He obviously never tried on 15 pairs in a changing room on a Saturday morning, eventually reaching that state most of us will have encountered which I call Denim Despair.

I am no fan of mutton dressed as lamb, but I think jeans can look good whatever your age.

Jeans shopping always—ALWAYS—has to be done in the flesh, unless you are repeat buying an exact style. Give yourself at least a couple of hours in a multi-brand store. Be prepared to try lots of brands, and to skip around on sizes, even within one brand.

There are two traditional approaches. One is to prioritize what best flatters your shape. The other is to look for what flatters your mind; that sense of who you are and how you want to present to the world. Because particular cuts of jeans have become so evocative of a time, a place, or a type of person. (That's why Saint Laurent's declaration is so far from the truth.) The once ubiquitous bootcut, for example, while flattering for a curvier shape, can these days look uncool. The still ubiquitous skinny is beginning to appear old-hat, too, and has also never been as flattering for many of us as we might like to think.

For me a new middle way is the best. I call it the mind-body

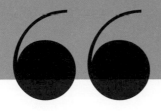

For somebody to dress well they have to feel what they are wearing.

—MIUCCIA PRADA

equation, in which you add together how you see yourself in your head with the realities of your body shape, and come up with an end result that works for both. It's a good rule of thumb for all shopping, but is particularly apposite for denim. As Miuccia Prada says, "For somebody to dress well they have to feel what they are wearing." But again, bear in mind that if you try to cover up a part of your body that you are not happy with, you will likely just make it look bigger.

WHAT SUITS WHO

Let's talk about the body part of the equation first. If you are petite and/or short in the leg you are going to be most flattered by a high-rise cropped style in a dark wash or black. If you are tall and/or long in the leg, look for a low-rise flare in the color of your choosing. A triangle will look best in a mid-rise straight leg in a medium stretch dark wash. If you are a column or an inverted triangle, go for a boyfriend jean in any wash. If you are a mix of two shapes then it's the shape of your bottom half that is relevant here. I am a triangle and an inverted triangle. Jeans-wise it's the first bit of this double act that matters, alas.

If you don't like the shape that suits you best—if it's not working for the mind bit of the equation—then some of the more recent denim tweaks have been designed for you. I like the aesthetic of a boyfriend for example, but they tend to paper-bag me around the waist and hips. The so-called girlfriend or slim boyfriend incarnation, which is sleeker, flatters me far more while still delivering an aesthetic I like.

Can't bring yourself to break it off with your skinnies? Try the relaxed skinny, which gives a little more room for maneuvering, or again the girlfriend/slim boyfriend. You can also consider switching between two styles, one more "mind," the other more "body." I now flip between the triangle-flattering straight-leg and my happy-place girlfriends.

Bear in mind though that jeans are one of the most problematic purchases around, environmentally speaking, using 2,115 gallons of water a pop and chemicals galore to make. G-Star Raw is changing things up with its Raw for the Planet range, which is made with 98 percent recycled water and a new indigo dye with 70 percent fewer chemicals.

THE DETAILS

As for the height of the waistband, the fashion pack will keep banging on about the high-rise—partly in response, I think, to all those years of low-rise styles—but for many of us, myself included, it won't work. That said, leave the low-rise for the super-tall, or super-skinny, too.

Factor in the effect of pocket size, shape, and placement, too: square back pockets that aren't tilted can also make a larger bottom look peachy. But if you are bigger, avoid fussy detailing on both pockets and belt loops.

Don't dismiss a modernizing frayed and/or stepped hem on an otherwise classic style, though go stealth not extreme. Or you could try some carefully chosen embellishment—a bit of diamanté here, a side stripe there. In either instance keep the rest of your look dialed down and/or classic. Slightly crazy jeans plus extremely sane tailored jacket is a combo that's hard to beat.

Dark washes tend to be more flattering on most people, and certainly more contemporary looking, though for the summer months white denim is back with a vengeance. Is white denim winter appropriate? I wouldn't wear it, but that doesn't mean you shouldn't. Though there is one denim rule I don't think should be broken: obvious fraying and/or holes. Not if you are over 25.

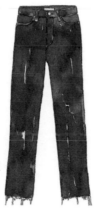

Don't dismiss a modernizing frayed and/or stepped hem on an otherwise classic style, though go stealth not extreme.

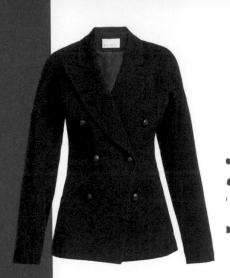

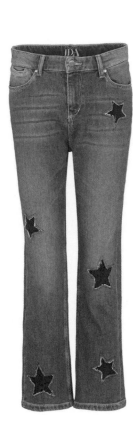

JACKET

+

EMBELLISHED
JEANS

*I love amped-up denim, but
I know to tread with care.
You want to see more actual
jean than embellishment.
Plus you should pair with
plain and/or chic pieces,
nothing else full-on. And
I mean nothing. Dialed-
back tailoring, or shirting.
Simple footwear.*

THE FASHION PACK'S FAVORITES

Whatever the style you go for, you tend to get what you pay for. Favorite brands with the fashion pack at a higher price point include Current Elliott, For All Mankind, Frame, James, MiH, and Paige. At a lower price point the picks are The Gap and Uniqlo.

Still not convinced? If you know your happy place is to be more elegant than casual, jeans may never be for you. But part of what denim endows is attitude. So why not wear another item of clothing in the same laid-back way? "Treat everything like your favorite pair of jeans," says the designer Roland Mouret. "A pencil skirt for example. It doesn't have to be challenging. It's reliable, comfortable, you can wear it with heels or flats, tuck a top in or wear it out." The non-jean jeans. You heard it here first.

Another route is to consider the new incarnation of denim. Think smartly tailored trousers—detail free, flat-fronted—that just happen to be chambray. Incredibly flattering. Think a genre-busting denim blazer. It will give an uptown ensemble downtown edge, and vice versa. And what was that ultimate uptown girl Carolina Herrera wearing when she told me she would never wear jeans again? A super-sharp denim shirt dress. Too old for jeans? Maybe. Too old for denim? Never. Forget that mutton dressed as lamb analogy; here was another species entirely, super-cool yet super-chic. Baaa.

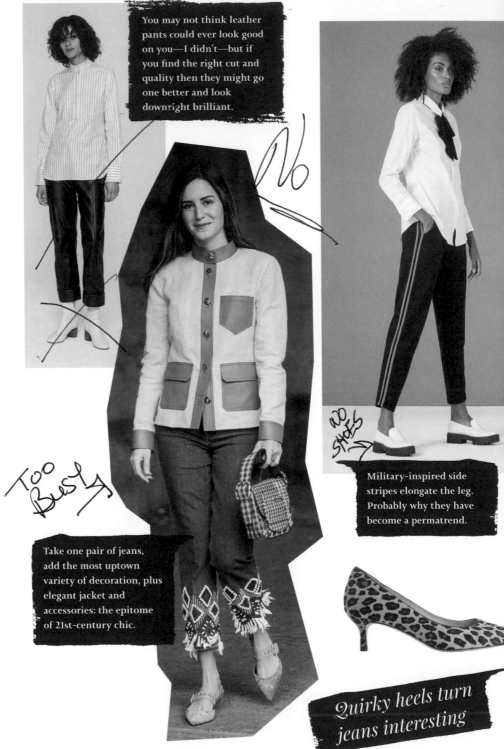

You may not think leather pants could ever look good on you—I didn't—but if you find the right cut and quality then they might go one better and look downright brilliant.

Military-inspired side stripes elongate the leg. Probably why they have become a permatrend.

Take one pair of jeans, add the most uptown variety of decoration, plus elegant jacket and accessories: the epitome of 21st-century chic.

Quirky heels turn jeans interesting

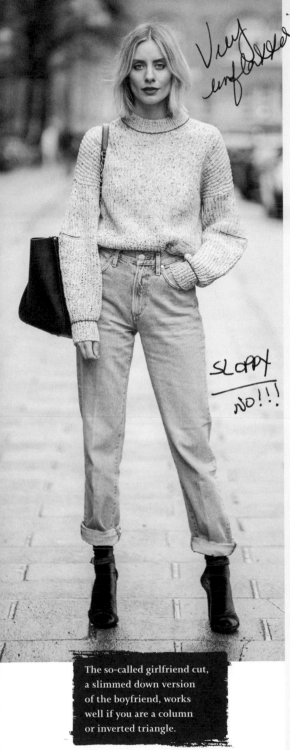

Very unflattering

TROUSERING IT

Pants and jeans can make you look effortlessly chic, and can be more straightforward to mix and match than a skirt. Those are two of the reasons why they are a default for the fashion pack, along with all the great options out there these days. Once you properly understand your body shape, and a few key details around cut and design, you will be able to find pants and jeans that really deliver for you.

SLOPPY
NO!!!

None of these look appropriate they look stupid actually! SLOPPY

The so-called girlfriend cut, a slimmed down version of the boyfriend, works well if you are a column or inverted triangle.

Wide—but not too wide—jeans can flatter columns, rectangles, and roundeds.

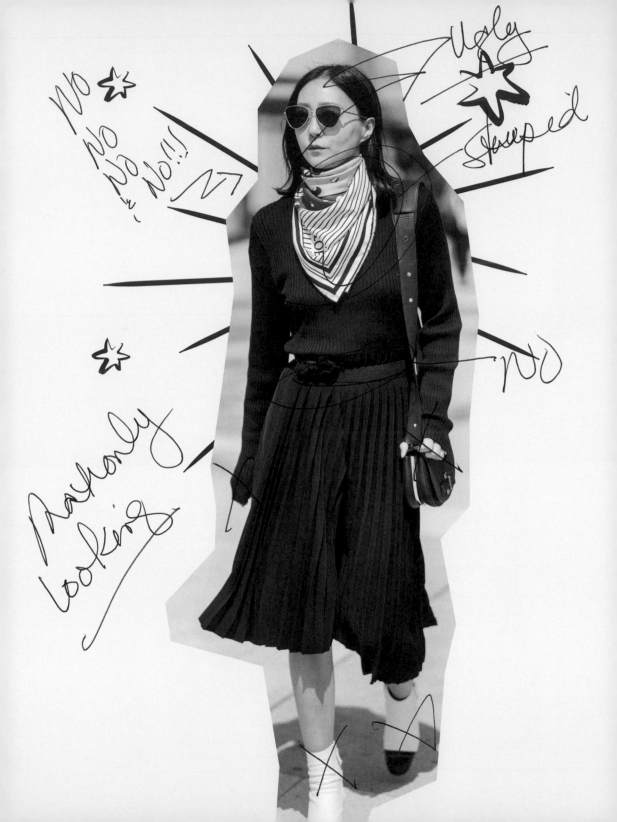

14

Look-
Lifters
and
Mad-Ons

HOW TO ORNAMENT YOUR WAY
TO INDIVIDUALITY

Just a single item can turn you from boring to brilliant, from lackluster to luscious. And it can be small. Small, but fabulous. Perhaps a great pair of earrings. Perhaps a slash of bright lipstick. Perhaps the twist of a hot-hued silk or fine-wool scarf. Perhaps nothing more than a belt. Perhaps a pair of embellished flats, or even—bear with me—socks.

I call them the look-lifters, those lone flourishes that have the ability to transform your appearance, to make you present *tout d'un coup* as fresher/cooler/brighter/younger, or all of the above. Honestly. It's all that's required.

You just need to make sure that flourish is properly noteworthy, rather than not-that-special. Those earrings and that scarf need to be genuinely beautiful, which doesn't have to mean expensive. That lipstick needs to be a look-at-me shade, not a librarian one. When it comes to socks I am not talking black ribbed—or maybe, but with a diamanté trim.

This one-hit-wonder route is the secret to the stylishness of many of the women I know on the front row. Sure, there are those who are always pushing the envelope head-to-toe, working a particular trend before it's even become recognized as such by the real world. But there are at least as many who wear a fairly simple, fairly unchanging get-up of the best quality they can afford, and then lift that look—which might otherwise appear almost dull in its dialed-down simplicity—by way of a tweak of something that is, to be frank, just a little bit showy.

The style diva Iris Apfel is another example of this methodology. "People think I wear spectacular outfits, but most of the time I don't," she once told me. "I believe in architectural clothes without any embellishment, so that I can embellish them in my own way."

THE BLING RING

Jewelry is the default *modus operandi* for the fashion pack, particularly earrings and necklaces. There's a reason why these two forms give the most bang for their buck, not that there needs to be

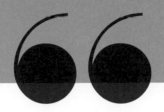

I believe in architectural clothes without any embellishment, so that I can embellish them in my own way.

—IRIS APFEL

much buck involved. That's because they sit next to the face, and it's the face that—on a basic animal level—human beings look at before anything else. So if you have a bit of *bijou* that twinkles nearby, well, to the state the obvious, the face, and particularly the eyes, look more twinkly, too. "A woman of my age needs diamonds near her face, to give sparkle," observes Lady Montdore, in Nancy Mitford's *Love in a Cold Climate*.

That's where pearls, as well as diamonds, come in. Or, if you are me, faux pearls and diamanté. (I am very much a costume jewelry kind of a girl. Luckily.) Whatever your skin tone, there is nothing better at flattering the complexion than the dazzle of a clear gemstone or the luster of a pearl, real or otherwise. I have some cluster earrings that are a combination of both, and however tired I am (or worse), that ear candy works like magic—like a facial, an eight-hour-sleep, and a hair-of-the-dog bloody mary combined.

There are essentially five ways to go when it comes to jewelry. Traditional, which tends to be modestly sized, and of a design your grandmother would recognize: pearl or diamond studs, or a string of pearls are obvious examples. Then there's the modernist-cum-minimalist—all sinuous curves of metal. Next up is the wide-ranging category encompassed by the term "ethnic" which, to generalize, looks to have been bought when you last went on a

Whatever your skin tone there is nothing better at flattering the complexion than the dazzle of a clear gemstone or the luster of a pearl.

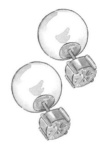

far-flung vacation, even if, in fact, you picked it up at a boutique or market stall just around the corner from your front door.

Finally there is what I call the Biggie Smalls variety, which comes in two different subsets; on the one hand luster that is little, on the other bling that is—you guessed it—big.

An unusual piece of vintage bling is, to my mind, unbeatable, but a predictable piece risks being, well, precisely that.

Of course there are overlaps within all these categories. In recent years, for example, there has developed a gorgeous new sub-category of modernist pearl designs, which combine all those time-immemorial complexion-enhancing pearl powers with the look-modernizing lines of a definitively 21st-century setting. Indeed, there has been such a wonderful flowering of creativity in jewelry design generally that there's never been a better time to adorn yourself— more than that, express yourself—via some carefully curated trinkets.

But which way to go? I would counsel against the uncompromisingly classicist route, as it can look old-fashioned. Though a slight retool would be just fine. Should you be up for an investment, Dior's double-pearl Tribales earrings, in which one pearl sits in front of the lobe, and another slightly larger one sits behind it are the perfect case in point. The boutique brand Wouters & Hendrix has countless more affordable variations on the theme of 21st-century pearl.

An unusual piece of vintage bling is, to my mind, unbeatable, but a predictable piece risks being, well, precisely that, and therefore not a look-lifter in the making. Ethnic can work, but take care. A sub-hippy-trail cliché can present as boringly as your grandmother's pearls. But a good piece—perhaps a necklace of

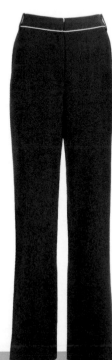

SIMPLE SHIRT

BLACK
TROUSERS

STATEMENT
EARRINGS

It can be as easy as a pair of earrings. That's all that's required to turn a classic look contemporary. Buy jewelry that's designed to flatter the complexion— pearls, real or otherwise, diamonds, ditto—retooled to appear up to date.

chunky stones in an unusual color, or a pair of intricately worked chandelier earrings—has true transformative power. What I would say when it comes to anything ethnic—clothing as well as bling—is only wear one thing at any time and keep the rest of your outfit plain and chic.

Tiny-tot trinkets have been a favorite with the fashion pack for years now. Indeed, they've reached the status of a permatrend. The trick is to layer up a lot that's little. Most fashion women now have ears that, courtesy of multi-piercings, look like constellations. If you don't like the idea of more than one piercing—which I don't—you can now buy assorted convincing fake alternatives, such as a so-called "ear crawler," which sits along the lobe, or an ear cuff, which is a hoop that you can position anywhere you choose along the outside edge of the ear.

At their neck, and on their wrists, these women stockpile myriad gold and silver fine threads and pendants, and—one style rule that has now been well and truly cast aside—show no compunction in mixing the two metals. The countless tiny rings on their fingers make me think of that "fine lady upon a white horse" in the well-known nursery rhyme; whether they too have bells on their toes I couldn't possibly comment. But what I do know is that the end result looks feminine, stylish, and ineffably now. It takes even a white shirt and black pants combo to another level. In short, it lifts it into a look.

What I would say when it comes to anything ethnic is only wear one thing at any time and keep the rest of your outfit plain and chic.

I am a member of the other jewelry contingent still out in force on the front row, though admittedly not as numerous. I like mine big. I think that's partly because I am big! My broad face suits some large statement earrings rather than anything too small. Though always check the weight before you buy, which is why I think it's best to shop in the flesh—literally—rather than online. Make sure they are of a weight your lobes will be happy with all day, even if you are only planning on wearing them for an evening. No one wants ear-candy that gets in the way of having a good time. The good news is that light-as-a-feather is easier than ever to track down. Beading, resin, and plastic all deliver stylistic heft without the literal variety. A heavy necklace can wreak havoc with your neck, too. Again, test before you buy.

If you are going Biggie, not Smalls, I would argue it's a case of earrings or necklace, not both. And bear in mind that a large necklace will dictate the kind of neckline you can wear. Which is why for me it's earrings almost every time.

SCARF CHIC

Not much of a jewelry person? Scarves are another way to look-lift. Color—possibly subtle, yet always unusual—is, along with an interesting pattern, the key to pulling off Peak Scarf. Though a warning: scarves can be tricky. Get it wrong and they look fussy and aging. But get it right and they look fabulous. Iris Apfel picked up her outfit-bespoking talents from her mother. "She worshipped at the altar of the accessory: she could do more tricks with a scarf than anyone I have ever met."

First off, it's scarf, or earrings, or necklace—not all three, although a scarf might just be acceptable with the aforementioned tiny jewelry. As Coco Chanel once said, "Before you leave the house, look in the mirror and take one thing off."

If you are wearing a scarf tied at the neck, make sure that said neck is long enough to pull it off. If you have a short neck, or even a medium-length one, a scarf can make it appear shorter. Some people can go the cravat approach, but I think it's cooler to wrap it around the neck several times then knot it at one side. Or you might want to consider the new-gen neckerchief, which is long and thin, rather than square, and specifically designed for the matter at hand. It adds interest to your look while leaving more of your neck on show, and thus minimizing any shortening effect.

The rules of bling-buying

My Irish potato-picker hands look better with a knuckle-duster or two I think. And from my three everyday rings I have learned the key lessons about jewelry purchasing.

1

That if you really, truly love a piece but think it is too expensive, buy it anyway—provided it is not bankruptcy-inducing, of course. Wear it every day, and you will never regret it. A broad dull gold band I bought 20 years ago for a sum that made me feel sick at the time (about $400) has, in terms of price per wear, proved to be one of the best-value items I own.

2

That an unusual piece will get you noticed time and again. I've lost count of how many people have complimented me on a 1950s watch-ring—yes, they used to be a thing— and a vintage Dior bobble ring, one of my luckiest junk-shop finds ever.

"

Before you leave
the house, look
in the mirror
and take one
thing off.

—COCO CHANEL

Don't wear a scarf like a shawl, unless you want to look like a fortune teller. And don't wear it long and loose over a dress. What makes a dress so flattering to the female figure is the unity of its lines: leave them to do their work. A neckerchief is the best approach with a dress if you insist.

Another acceptable option is to wear a scarf draped lean and loose with a jacket, either peeping out beneath the collar line, or sitting on top, next to the lapels, or even—if the scarf is thin enough—under them.

The most foolproof way to add in a feminine flutter of scarf-liness is to tie one to the handle of your handbag: it's a perfect way to jazz up some otherwise sensible leather goods. Though I would argue that a popping or a patterned handbag is another look-lifter in the making.

BELT UP

Fashion stylists love belts, because they are an easy way not only to lift a look, but also to change a silhouette. "Little things, like a belt or some earrings, can switch up your look instantly," says red-carpet pro Rebecca Corbin-Murray. "You don't need to have ten dresses. You can have one or two." A single unwaisted black dress becomes several if you wear it not only loose but with a narrow belt or a wide one. Add in a colored and/or embellished belt and

225

The most foolproof way to add in a feminine flutter of scarf-liness is to tie one to the handle of your handbag.

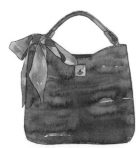

you have yet more options, and have turned said dress into one of the hardest-working items in your wardrobe.

Just bear in mind your body shape when it comes to belts. If you are an hourglass—neat or full—then sally forth and belt away. If you are a triangle or an inverted triangle, you need to skim your larger section, and emphasize your smaller, to add overall balance to your silhouette. Similarly, a column should add emphasis to the shoulders and/or hips. Those who are a rectangle or rounded shape should proceed with caution, if it all. (See Chapter 1)

FANCY FLATS

It probably goes without saying that shoes are the ultimate look-lifter. Cinderella's slippers certainly got her noticed, and they can do the same for us. What's changed is that we, unlike her, have the option to wear look-at-me shoes we can run in as well as look like a princess in. Flats are no longer for frumps. Indeed, some of the fanciest footwear these days comes minus a heel, but with the addition of countless other things, from diamanté to sequins. And some sneakers are so blinged-out as to dazzle like the Crown Jewels. So you don't need to save footwear-related look-lifting for special occasions only. You can pull it off while sprinting after the bus, or doing the supermarket shopping.

You don't need to save footwear-related look-lifting for special occasions only.

And have you thought about socks? Really! Quirky socks have become quite the thing in Fashion Land in recent years. These are more than just a look-lifter. They are a veritable mad-on; one of those slightly crazy flourishes that adds just the right amount of lunatic edge to an otherwise sane ensemble.

It is the front-row rise of the cropped pant—surprisingly flattering, whatever your height—that has brought with it an

Shady character

Another popular mad-on is a pair of bonkers sunglasses. Until I found myself on the front row many years ago I—like most of you, I imagine— picked sensible shades. Frame-wise it had to be tortoiseshell, or maybe black or metal. Shape- wise, nothing too large or too dramatic. And I assumed that as I got older my choices would become even more restrained. Then suddenly I found myself surrounded by women in their fifties and sixties who off-set their considerable poise with glasses that, by non-fashion- standards, looked certifiable: mad colors and shapes. Once I had got over my initial amazement I realized those glasses made them look younger, made them look cooler, and didn't, to my surprise, make them look deranged. Since then silly shades have become a favorite mad on of mine; another effortless way to look-lift, sunshine permitting.

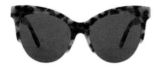

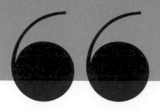

Little things, like a belt or some earrings, can switch up your look instantly. You don't need to have ten dresses. You can have one or two.

—REBECCA CORBIN-MURRAY

obsession with hot-to-trot hosiery worthy of a Regency dandy. They usually get worn with lace ups, as you might expect— perhaps in a pretty pattern and/or with an embellished edge— but the new development is stocking-socks that are paired with feminine flats, kitten heels, or platform sandals.

It took me a while to get my head around the whole notion. I am a slow-adopter among the fashion pack. But now I am a firm fan.

So dismiss the notion as nonsensical if you must, but the stocking-sock could work wonders for you, too, promise. With a skirt or dress this is, admittedly, what we in fashion call a "strong look." (Yet a killer one all the same.) But with those cut-off pants it is just the right side of cool. A flash of fishnet-socked ankle has garnered me countless compliments far away from planet fashion.

66

A flash of fishnet-socked ankle has garnered me countless compliments far away from planet fashion.

When I met up with red-carpet-stylist Elizabeth Saltzman recently, she was wearing a navy sweater and pants, plus a cream silk t-shirt. But on one finger was a ball-breaker of a ring in the shape of a turtle. That jewelry was proper stuff—emeralds and diamonds, don't you know—but it could just as easily have been costume, and she would still have looked like a million dollars. And what did she compliment me on? My fishnet socks. Not in the same stratosphere, but they did the same job. Look and learn from both of us. Then look-lift or mad-on accordingly.

Fishnet socks have become an interest-adding go-to for the fashion pack—not that zebra print mules need any help in that department.

The idea of wearing mad sunglasses might seem, well, mad. Not necessarily. A shape and color that's out-there can render you instantly in.

The plainest of ensembles is transformed by a colorful bag and shoes.

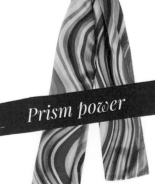

Prism power

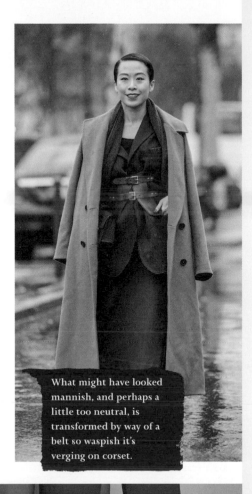

BIG LITTLE TWEAKS

It doesn't take much to transform a look. The canniest shoppers put the legwork into finding pieces that really suit them and that will last, then reinvent them over and again with accessories. Shoes, bags, belts, jewelry, scarves, sunglasses. This stuff is fun to buy and fun to wear. Especially now that there are so many brilliant options to choose from. And you don't have to sacrifice on practicality either. So enjoy!

What might have looked mannish, and perhaps a little too neutral, is transformed by way of a belt so waspish it's verging on corset.

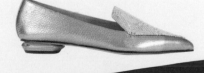

Twinkle toes

It was only a matter of time before the ever-fashionable and flattering cropped pant trend prompted the front row to fall in love with the ankle sock. Buy quirky and your hosiery will transform even the most sensible footwear.

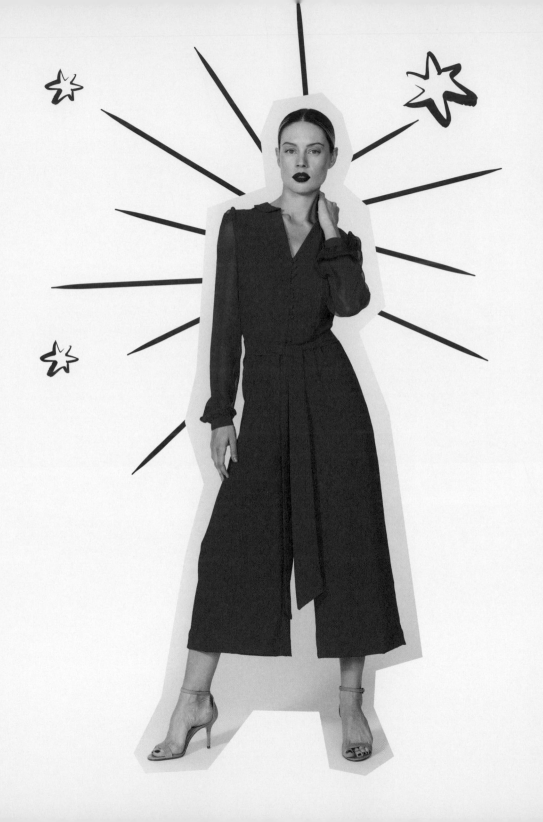

15

Peak
Chic

HOW TO GET EVENT
DRESSING RIGHT

Most of life takes place at middling altitude. It's hill and dale stuff at best. Not a mountainscape. Weekdays follow weekends follow weekdays. The work-play seesaw, er, seesaws, and in so doing spends at least as much time hovering in that no man's land that is not quite work but is definitely not play; the one that encompasses everything from a trip to the farmers' market to parents' evenings.

It's what we wear to all of the above that shapes our wardrobe, and rightly so. Yet we spend at least as much time and money—often more—on the clothes we wear for those rare moments when life turns lofty. When—courtesy of a wedding, or a big birthday, or a friend selflessly deciding to throw a really great party for no reason whatsoever—we are suddenly existing, and dressing, at an entirely different elevation.

It is this very point of difference that makes it easy to go astray. Occasionwear. Even the word sounds frumpy. And that's how occasionwear can often end up looking: old-fashioned, overdone, not very "you." The point is not suddenly to present like someone else entirely, especially when that someone is your father's spinster aunt. Rather you want to look like the best possible version of yourself. So you need to wear what you love, what you know suits you from trial and—hopefully not too much—error.

BE TRUE TO YOU *Occasionwear*

In short, if dresses aren't your thing, don't wear one. If you can't walk in heels, don't try to. If you feel awkward in a hat, now is not the time to start attempting to convince yourself otherwise. Think of the kind of outfit that both flatters you and puts you at your ease—the two usually go hand in hand—and invest in the best possible version you can find.

Shop as you normally would, in other words, only perhaps with an eye to having a little more fun with color and/or pattern. But bear in mind that this is the kind of occasion when you are more likely than usual to be photographed. Follow the advice of Samantha Cameron who, as a former British Prime Minister's

"

Nothing too fussy, because it just looks more fussy in pictures.

—SAMANTHA CAMERON

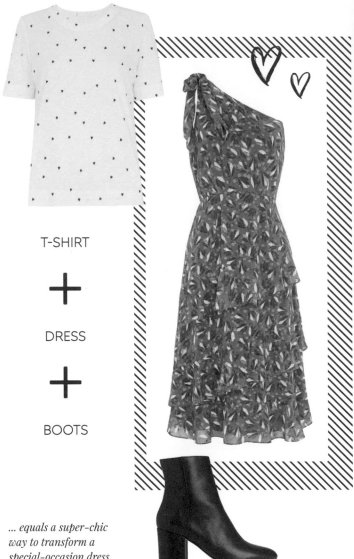

T-SHIRT

+

DRESS

+

BOOTS

... equals a super-chic way to transform a special-occasion dress into something you are happy wearing seven days a week.

wife, had to learn fast what did and didn't work on camera. "Nothing too fussy," she says, "because it just looks more fussy in pictures."

Above all, never buy anything that you aren't confident you will wear over and again back in your sea-level existence. You've heard of shelf life. Start factoring in wardrobe life. However divine a particular dress is, if it's a one-event wonder it's no good to anyone. Who has got the money, not to mention the hanging space, to fritter away like that? Never buy a fashion one-night stand. Buy a love-affair-in-waiting.

But don't use this as an excuse to shop boringly, to pedestrianize your fashion life yet further. Instead, look at things through the other end of the style telescope. If you love a floaty floral dress, if it makes you feel like a princess for the day, yet you somehow only ever wear one if you are invited to a wedding, ask yourself why. And change things up accordingly. Why not make every day an occasion? Or at least a couple of days a month? Your clothes can do that for you. That is the power of fashion.

Never buy a fashion one-night stand. Buy a love-affair-in-waiting.

Buy that dress you have fallen in love with for said wedding. Then, once you've shaken out the confetti, wear it for coffee with friends. For a shopping trip. For dinner with your partner. Sure, add in an everyday edge courtesy of sneakers or stompy boots, with perhaps a t-shirt underlayer, or a bomber or vest on top, but WEAR IT. And *keep on wearing it.*

Life doesn't have to be lived in Monday-to-Friday suits and Saturday-to-Sunday jeans. Make peak chic a more regular occurrence than a handful of times a year. Enjoy that feeling of high-altitude specialness without having to wait for a gilt-edged invite. Get your friends in on the program. Have dress-up dates, in which you all agree to go the extra style mile. It's such fun.

FUN + FUSS = FNUSS

Fun. That's a key word. Parties and weddings are supposed to be fun, and the same should go for the build-up. By all means fuss in advance about your outfit—I know I do—but make sure that the fussing is also fun. Fnuss. It's one of my favorite activities. There is nothing I relish more than to fnuss over my outfit in the run-up to a big bash.

Thankfully there is more opportunity to fnuss than ever before. It's now easier—and more affordable—to dress gorgeously. There are so many great options out there at every price point. And all those former fashion unicorns, such as dresses with long sleeves and flattering mid-calf skirts, are two-a-penny. Plus, the rules as to what is or isn't acceptable for a woman to wear no longer apply. However posh the engagement, these days it's fine to wear trousers, as long as they're killer. And the best rule-retirement of all is that dressing up no longer has to involve discomfort. Indeed, to my mind it is positively *verboten*. You look your best when you look at ease. Shop accordingly.

THE DRESSY DRESS

I think there are three main ways to look modern, not matronly, when a boldface event beckons.

For the evening it's hard to go wrong with a little black dress, though I would consider it a mite too funereal for nuptials. The LBD is a codification of chic, and for anything evening it's hard to beat. Which isn't to say it's impossible to get wrong. Too short or too tight is a no-go. And don't make the mistake of over-complicating the add-ons. The LBD works because of its simplicity. Which will be undone *tout d'un coup* if you mess up its clean lines. Pick one elaborate and/or colorful flourish, maybe two—perhaps your earrings, or necklace, or shoes, but

However posh the engagement, these days it's fine to wear trousers, as long as they're killer.

The LBD decree

One of the many great things about the little black dress is that it's hard to get wrong. But, alas, it's not impossible. And some approaches are definitely more right than others.

1

Make sure it's not too little. Overly short or tight is a surefire way to turn classy into catastrophe.

2

If you go for a classic style of frock, make sure to change it up with one or two modernizing accessories. Better still, look for flourishes that are just that little bit surprising.

3

If you choose a style that is ultra-contemporary or full-on in terms of detailing, keep everything else dialed down.

definitely not all three—and keep everything else dialed down (see pp.62–63).

Next up is the floaty dress, which might be a print (floral or otherwise), or a plain (bright or subdued), and which will serve you at every event imaginable. This is a genre that has been revolutionized in recent years, to the eternal benefit of womankind.

There's a floaty dress out there that will render every single one of us the belle of the ball. You just have to find it. Pick a color you love, pick a neckline and cut that suits. The new multifariousness of fashion means that all options are out there, every season. You will by now be unsurprised to learn that I would sneak a jumpsuit or co-ords iteration of both the sleek/black and floaty/colorful options here. They deliver everything that a great dress does.

Favor sleeves by all means—there are more good sleeved than sleeveless styles around now—but don't rule out buying sleeveless and adding a pretty top layer, be it an embellished cardigan or a luxe bomber.

Indeed, new-gen cover-ups can be a great way to ensure you look youthful. Other options include the shearling vest, the cropped cape, and the sleeveless coat. Proceed cautiously with the bolero: you can end up looking like you are due on stage at the Royal Opera House. And steer clear of a shawl unless you have a sartorial skill set to match Kate Moss's.

> **Don't rule out buying sleeveless and adding a pretty top layer, be it an embellished cardigan or a luxe bomber.**

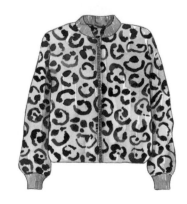

You might also like to consider Spanx's Arm Tights as an option, a stockingesque arm-covering which has become popular with the less triceps-happy denizens of the red carpet. "Great for anyone who doesn't like their arms," says celebrity stylist Elizabeth Saltzman.

SKIRTING THE ISSUE

As for skirt length, find your sweet spot—the point at which your legs look their best—using the towel test detailed in the Bodymapping chapter (see p.34). For many of us a mid-calf cut is the most flattering, because it draws attention to what remains, whatever your age, that most coltish of body parts, the ankle. For the petite it may be somewhere around the knee, that extra flesh providing length and height to your look. Whatever your shape or size, a longer cut with a leg-flashing slit can deliver the best of both worlds.

And, still on the subject of skirts, don't dismiss that asymmetric hem, which can effortlessly update an otherwise classic dress (see pp.103–104). Just make sure to look for a hem whose dips and dives are stealthy rather than full-on swallow.

SUITS YOU

Tailoring. Gosh, it's hard to beat a tuxedo suit. Again, not black for a daytime wedding. You don't want to look as if you have turned up at the ceremony for another type of event entirely. But there are now so many great colored takes, from low-key pastels to party brights. And black could work brilliantly for an evening or black-tie wedding. Plus—along with preternaturally stylish cream or white—for anything that isn't a nuptials. Whatever color you go for, you might also consider a twin-hue, with a contrast shade for lapel and buttons. Utterly classic, but original, too. There's something about those sharp tailored lines that paradoxically draw out a woman's femininity at least as much as a floral dress. The alchemy at work may be different, but the end result is a variation on the theme of womanly wonderfulness.

What lies beneath

Rebecca Corbin-Murray is a stylist whose job it is to pour some of the world's most fabulous women into some of the world's most fabulous dresses, and even they need Spanx, she tells me. "I put everyone in Spanx. It always looks better." Which cut to buy? "You need an arsenal" she laughs. "And I mean an arsenal. Different lengths and coming up to different heights." Personally, I am a fan of the styles you can wear with your own bra, in particular the mid-thigh bodysuit range.

When it comes to that bra make sure whatever you wear isn't visible. Bodas nude styles are good, and for a backless, strapless option I have been impressed by Fashion Forms' Go Bare style, which goes up to an E cup size, is a stick on that actually sticks on, and can be used up to 25 times. You want stealth panties, too: Commando's seamless styles—available in nude and black, in a variety of cuts—will do the job nicely.

A big, blowsy corsage—fresh or synthetic—feminizes the look further. Keep your underlayer soft and, ideally, silken or crispest cotton, be it a shirt, blouse, or tee, either white or cream, or in a delicious complementary hue. If your jacket or neckline isn't too low, and you are feeling slinky, you might even go for just a bra underneath. *Yes! Bustier is Gorg!*

Whichever take on the tuxedo suit you go for, it will translate effortlessly for life in the real world, be it the whole package for the office, or just the tux jacket with jeans for a relaxed weekend meet-up. Maybe think twice about that corsage. Though, on reflection, maybe not.

FOOTLOOSE

There are no rules when it comes to footwear either. OK, maybe one. That you should be comfortable. (Sound familiar?) After all, so many big events are looooong, and—in the summer months— may encompass some off-roading. Make sure you are shod accordingly. You don't want a day to feel like a lifetime. You don't want to have to sit down on the job.

Thankfully, fashion fell in love with the embellished flat a while back, and is now similarly besotted with heels so dinky as to be almost fit for running a marathon. The industry has christened them nano-heels. They might also be called almost-flats, that's how comfortable they are, but they still add a feminine edge that is perfect for a special bash—provided it's not a grass-bash of course, in which case stick to flats, a wedge, platform, or a chunky mid-heel.

More comfortable still would be a pair of embellished sneakers, or even some plain white ones, as long as white is what they still are. For a big event, I would only wear a brand new pair. Sneakers can work well both with that floaty dress, or that sharp pantsuit, though generally not with an LBD (unless it has a long, full skirt). Even at the flashiest fashion do it's rare for there not to be at least one woman in whiter than white clean Adidas Stan Smiths. It's for you to weigh up the nature of the event, and the type of guest list, although, in actuality, it's often more about the latter rather than the former. It's the attitude of your inviters and fellow invitees that will above all determine what is and isn't deemed acceptable. You know better than anyone what that is. But never be afraid to find your own happy place. It's your opinion that is always the most important.

HATS 'N' HAIR

Headgear-wise, only wear a hat if you like a hat, as discussed. And be wary of the deceptively named fascinator, which can be one of the least fascinating, most aging items of attire around. It is hard to go wrong with a classic style like a Panama, perhaps pared back, perhaps with some tweaking in the form of a colored band, some embroidery, or a flower or two.

If you want something more extravagant, it's easiest to start your outfit from the hat, rather than vice versa. Consider both your frame and your face shape. A hat should never be wider than the shoulders, and if you are petite, a good option is to pick a small base with upstanding feathers or quills for height. If your face is rounded—the trickiest shape to make work with millinery—a slanting style can add length. Go into a shop and try lots of options on. It can be difficult to figure out what really suits you. Get someone to take pictures from different angles. Go home, think about it, then go back. You know the drill by now. And as with everything else you buy and wear, make sure your hat is comfortable, make sure you can last all day in it. Otherwise you will buy it and not wear it ever again.

Consider both your frame and your face shape. A hat should never be wider than the shoulders.

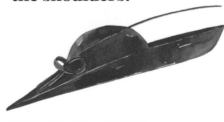

Treat yourself to a blow-out if you are not wearing a hat, but ask for loose and laid-back, not uptight and aging. Again, keep make-up minimalist. Let your skin shine through, whatever your age. Burnish it, don't cover it up. And go for eyes or lips, not both.

What is nonnegotiable when it comes to lips is that, when that circled date finally comes around, you smile, smile, smile. Which you will be doing anyway courtesy of all that lovely fnuss, and the glorious end results.

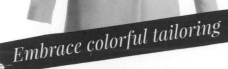

Embrace colorful tailoring

246

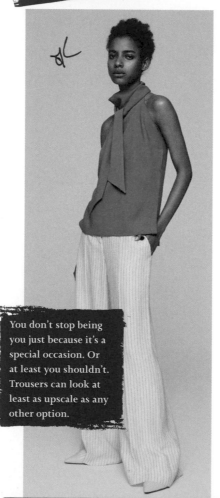

Three things to learn from this look. That, done right, separates can out-glamour the opposition. That, more specifically, a white shirt can achieve the same. And that a smile is always the most important accessory.

You don't stop being you just because it's a special occasion. Or at least you shouldn't. Trousers can look at least as upscale as any other option.

If the prospect of wearing a hat gives you a thrill, enjoy it! Shop for the hat first. Then find the outfit.

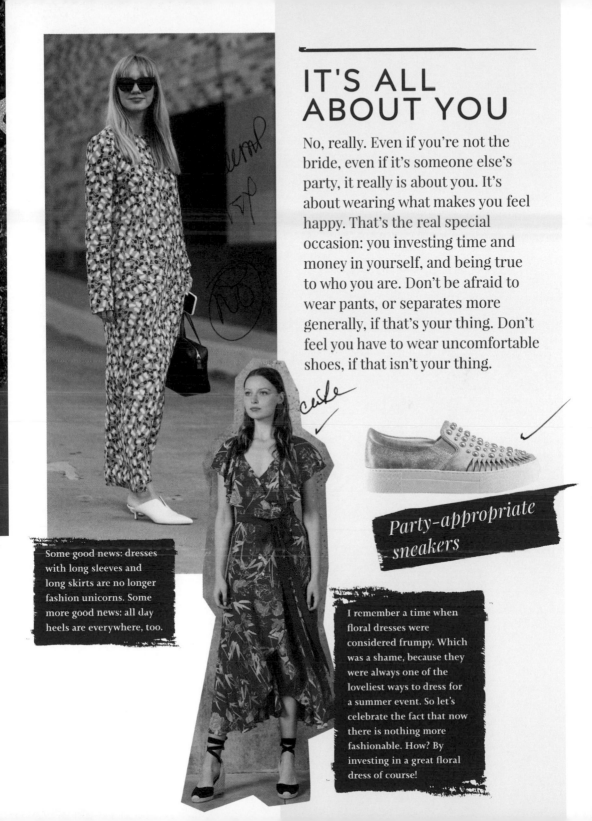

IT'S ALL ABOUT YOU

No, really. Even if you're not the bride, even if it's someone else's party, it really is about you. It's about wearing what makes you feel happy. That's the real special occasion: you investing time and money in yourself, and being true to who you are. Don't be afraid to wear pants, or separates more generally, if that's your thing. Don't feel you have to wear uncomfortable shoes, if that isn't your thing.

Party-appropriate sneakers

Some good news: dresses with long sleeves and long skirts are no longer fashion unicorns. Some more good news: all day heels are everywhere, too.

I remember a time when floral dresses were considered frumpy. Which was a shame, because they were always one of the loveliest ways to dress for a summer event. So let's celebrate the fact that now there is nothing more fashionable. How? By investing in a great floral dress of course!

INDEX

PICTURE CREDITS

The publisher would like to thank the following for their kind permission to reproduce their photographs:

(Key: a-above; b-below/bottom; c-center; f-far; l-left; r-right; t-top)

10 News Licensing: Sarah Cresswell / The Times Magazine. **18 123RF.com:** Ekaterina Bychkova (stars). **Baukjen:** (c). **19 123RF.com:** Anna Babii (b). **27 123RF.com:** astrozombie (t). **31 123RF.com:** astrozombie (t). **Essentiel Antwerp:** (bl). **The Fold:** (cr). **34 123RF.com:** Ekaterina Bychkova. **36-37 123RF.com:** astrozombie (brush strokes). **36 Baukjen:** (tr, bc). **Boden:** (tl) **Donna Ida / Kate Gorbunova:** Kate Gorbunova (bl). **37 Getty Images:** Daniel Zuchnik (bl). **Marks & Spencer:** (br). **Me + Em:** (tl). **38 123RF. com:** Ekaterina Bychkova (stars). **Getty Images:** Christian Vierig (c). **39 123RF.com:** Anna Babii (b). **45 123RF.com:** astrozombie (tl). **46 123RF.com:** Ekaterina Bychkova. **50 123RF.com:** astrozombie (t). **Baukjen:** (cl). **John Lewis:** (cr). **Russell & Bromley:** (clb). **54 Chinti & Parker:** (bl). **Getty Images:** Christian Vierig (tl); Daniel Zuchnik (tr). **54-55 123RF.com:** astrozombie (brush strokes). **55 Luisa Cerano / Esther Heesch @ MODELWERK:** (br). **Marks & Spencer:** (l). **56 123RF.com:** Ekaterina Bychkova (stars). **Getty Images:** Elisabetta Villa / Stringer (c). **57 123RF.com:** Anna Babii (b). **63 123RF. com:** astrozombie (tl). **DeMellier:** (br). **Kurt Geiger:** (crb). **Marks & Spencer:** (tr). **MATCHESFASHION.COM:** Dolce & Gabbana (cl). **NARS:** (cra). **64 123RF.com:** Ekaterina Bychkova (tr). **Boden:** (bc). **MATCHESFASHION.COM:** Racil (bl, br). **67 123RF.com:** astrozombie (tl); Anna Babii (cr); Galina Nikolaeva (dots). **Baukjen:** (cla). **Beulah:** (crb). **68 123RF.com:** Ekaterina Bychkova. **72 Getty Images:** Christian Vierig (tr). **MATCHESFASHION.COM:** Rockins (tl). **Me + Em:** (bl). **72-73 123RF.com:** astrozombie (brush strokes). **73 Essentiel Antwerp:** (bc). **Luisa Cerano / Esther Heesch @MODELWERK:** (bl, br). **The Kooples:** (tl). **74 123RF.com:** Ekaterina Bychkova (stars). **Getty Images:** Edward Berthelot (c). **75 123RF.com:** Anna Babii (b). **81 123RF.com:** astrozombie (tl). **84 Donna Ida / Kate Gorbunova:** Kate Gorbunova (c). **Luisa Cerano / Esther Heesch @MODELWERK:** (l). **Net-A-Porter:** Dinosaur Designs (tc). **84-85 123RF.com:** astrozombie (brush strokes). **85 Chinti & Parker:** Tom Mitchell (bc). **Me + Em:** (tl). **Net-A-Porter:** Alice & Olivia (br). **86 123RF.com:** Ekaterina Bychkova (stars). **Getty Images:** Melodie Jeng (c). **87 123RF.com:** Anna Babii (b). **90 123RF.com:** Ekaterina Bychkova. **93 123RF.com:** Ekaterina Bychkova (tr). **96 Getty Images:** Christian Vierig (br); Daniel Zuchnik (tl). **Net-A-Porter:** J Crew (tr). **96-97 123RF.com:** astrozombie (brush strokes). **97 Anna Walker:** (br). **Marks & Spencer:** (bl). **The Kooples:** (tl). **98 123RF.com:** Ekaterina Bychkova (stars). **Getty Images:** Kirstin Sinclair (c). **99 123RF.com:** Anna Babii (b). **106 123RF.com:** astrozombie (tl); Galina Nikolaeva (dots); Anna Babii (cb, tc). **Libby London:** (tr). **Russell & Bromley:** (bl). **108 Getty Images:** Kirstin Sinclair (r); Timur Emek (l). **Kurt Geiger:** (tr). **108-109 123RF. com:** astrozombie (brush strokes). **109 Primrose Park / Linnéa Berzén / Amy Hallam:** (bl). **Rixo London:** (tl). **Rock The Jumpsuit:** (bc). **110 123RF.com:** Ekaterina Bychkova (stars). **Getty Images:** Ben Hider (c). **111 123RF.com:** Anna Babii (b). **121 123RF.com:** astrozombie (tl); Anna Babii (ca). **Baukjen:** (cra). **Dorothee Schumacher:** (cla). **MATCHESFASHION.COM:** Raey (bc). **122 Beulah:** Matthew Eades (l). **Getty Images:** Jacopo Raule (r). **Rena Sala:** Laura Lombardi (tl). **122-123 123RF.com:** astrozombie (brush strokes). **123 Getty Images:** Christian Vierig (l). **MATCHESFASHION.COM:** Rochas (bc). **Me + Em:** (br). **124 123RF.com:** Ekaterina Bychkova (stars). **Filippa K:** (c). **125 123RF.com:** Anna Babii (b). **130 People Tree:** (br). **131 123RF.com:** Ekaterina Bychkova. **135 Maison de Mode:** Alepel / Saved You A Seat (bl). **136 Filippa K:** (bl). **137 People Tree:** (tl). **138 123RF.com:** Ekaterina Bychkova

251

(stars). **Getty Images:** Melodie Jeng (c). **139 123RF.com:** Anna Babii (b). **146 123RF.com:** Ekaterina Bychkova. **148 Getty Images:** Christian Vierig (l, r). **MATCHESFASHION. COM:** Christian Louboutin (tl). **148-149 123RF.com:** astrozombie (brush strokes). **149 Getty Images:** Christian Vierig (br). **LK Bennett:** (bl, crb). **The Kooples:** (tl). **150 123RF.com:** Ekaterina Bychkova (stars). **Donna Ida / Kate Gorbunova:** Kate Gorbunova (c). **151 123RF.com:** Anna Babii. **154 123RF.com:** astrozombie (tl). **LK Bennett:** (tr, crb). **Marks & Spencer:** (cl). **159 123RF.com:** astrozombie (tl). **Boden:** (bc, br). **Essentiel Antwerp:** (c). **Jigsaw:** (ca, cra). **Whistles:** (cr). **162 Essentiel Antwerp:** (tr). **Getty Images:** Christian Vierig (br); Venturelli (l). **162-163 123RF.com:** astrozombie (brush strokes). **163 Rixo London:** (br). **SET:** (tl). **Whistles:** (bl). **164 123RF.com:** Ekaterina Bychkova (stars). **Getty Images:** Christian Vierig (c). **165 123RF.com:** Anna Babii. **168 123RF.com:** Ekaterina Bychkova. **171 123RF.com:** astrozombie (tl). **LK Bennett:** (bc). **Marks & Spencer:** (cla). **Me + Em:** (cr). **176 Essentiel Antwerp:** (bl). **Getty Images:** Christian Vierig (tl, tr). **Luisa Cerano / Esther Heesch @MODELWERK:** (br). **176-177 123RF.com:** astrozombie (brush strokes). **177 Adidas:** (cb). **Me + Em:** (l, br). **178 123RF. com:** Ekaterina Bychkova (stars). **Getty Images:** Christian Vierig (c). **179 123RF.com:** Anna Babii. **185 123RF.com:** Ekaterina Bychkova. **186 123RF.com:** astrozombie (t); Anna Babii (clb). **Baukjen:** (bc). **LK Bennett:** (tr). **Whistles:** (tl, cl, cb, cr). **189 123RF.com:** astrozombie (tl). LK Bennett: (bc). MATCHESFASHION.COM: Gucci (cla); Sara Battaglia (cl). **Me + Em:** (tr). **Whistles:** (br). **192 Getty Images:** Matthew Sperzel (l); Mireya Acierto (r). **Marks & Spencer:** (bc). **Whistles:** (ca). **192-193 123RF.com:** astrozombie (brush strokes). **193 Baukjen:** (l). **Hobbs:** (br). **LK Bennett:** (cr). **194 123RF.com:** Ekaterina Bychkova (stars). **Getty Images:** Christian Vierig (c). **195 123RF.com:** Anna Babii. **199 123RF.com:** Ekaterina Bychkova. **203 123RF.com:** astrozombie (tl); Anna Babii (crb); Galina Nikolaeva (dots). **Jigsaw:** (cla). **LK Bennett:** (cb). **204 123RF.com:** astrozombie (tl). **210 123RF.com:** astrozombie (tl); Anna Babii (t); Galina Nikolaeva (dots). **Donna Ida / Kate Gorbunova:** (cr). **MATCHESFASHION.COM:** Raey (cla). **212 Baukjen:** (tr). **Getty Images:** Christian Vierig (c). **LK Bennett:** (crb). **Me + Em:** (tl). **212-213 123RF.com:** astrozombie (brush strokes). **213 Getty Images:** Christian Vierig (l). **Me + Em:** (br). 214 123RF.com: Ekaterina Bychkova (stars). **Getty Images:** Christian Vierig (c). **215 123RF.com:** Anna Babii. **220 123RF.com:** astrozombie (tl); Anna Babii (tc); Galina Nikolaeva (dots). **Baukjen:** (cla). **Tibi:** (bc). **Wouters & Hendrix:** (cra). **223 123RF.com:** Ekaterina Bychkova. **227 123RF.com**: Ekaterina Bychkova (tr). **Vow London:** (bc). **230 Getty Images:** Edward Berthelot (tl, tr); Vanni Bassetti (cl). **Paul Smith:** (bc). **230-231 123RF.com:** astrozombie (brush strokes). **231 Getty Images:** Edward Berthelot (tl). **Happy Socks:** (bl). **Nicholas Kirkwood Beya Loafers:** (cr). **232 123RF.com:** Ekaterina Bychkova (stars). **Rock The Jumpsuit:** (c). **233 123RF.com:** Anna Babii. **236 123RF.com:** astrozombie (tl); Anna Babii (cra, cra/Hearts). **LK Bennett:** (cb). **Whistles:** (cla, cr). **239 123RF.com:** Ekaterina Bychkova. **242 123RF.com:** Ekaterina Bychkova. **246 Getty Images:** Mike Marsland (tr). **MATCHESFASHION.COM:** Racil (tl). **Max Mara at Fenwicks:** (br). **Me + Em:** (bl). **246-247 123RF.com:** astrozombie (brush strokes). **247 Beulah:** Matthew Eades (bc). **Getty Images:** Christian Vierig (tl). **Russell & Bromley:** (cr)

All other images © Dorling Kindersley
For further information see: www.dkimages.com

ACKNOWLEDGMENTS

For their expertise and inspiration I would like to thank the fashion professionals I have referred to in these pages: Emmanuelle Alt, Iris Apfel, Christiane Arp, Anna Berkeley, Thea Bregazzi, Samantha Cameron, Maria Grazia Chiuri, Alexa Chung, Rebecca Corbin-Murray, Domenico Dolce, Rebecca Earley, Stefano Gabbana, Felicity Green, Demna Gvasalia, Clare Hornby, Carolina Herrera, Tommy Hilfiger, Annabel Hodin, Norma Kamali, Michael Kors, Christian Louboutin, Roland Mouret, Miuccia Prada, Elizabeth Saltzman, Justin Thornton, Anna Valentine, Donatella Versace, Diane von Furstenberg, and Dilys Williams.

For making the production of these pages an entirely happy experience I would like to thank Mary-Clare, Kathryn, Saffron, Vivienne, the rest of the team at Dorling Kindersley, and Rachael.

For transforming my working life into being about my words as much as other people's, I would like to thank John, Emma, Grace and, above all, Nicola.

For knowing there is more to life—to me—than clothes, I would like to thank my beloved parents, Rosemary and Peter, and my dear sister, Fran. Not forgetting my other, self-made family, especially Sarah and Geoff, the Emma's, the Rachel's, plus Charlotte, Jenny, Justine, Lisa, Robin, and Wendy.

DK would like to thank Rachael Dove for picture research, Philippa Nash for design assistance, Marie Lorimer for the index, Constance Novis for proofreading, and The Society of Authors as the Literary Representative of the Estate of Rosamond Lehmann.

ABOUT THE AUTHOR

As Fashion Director of *The Times* of London **Anna Murphy** divides her time between the fantasy realm of the front row and what, to her mind, is the true fashion frontline: the brands that deliver clothes for the real world. How to track down the right pieces for your life, your shape; how to look effortlessly stylish and contemporary; and how to do it without paying a fortune—that's what Anna sets out to nail in her writing. Not to mention in her own shopping!

Retail therapy in the most literal sense, that's Anna's thing. And after more years than she would care to admit on the fashion circuit—first as Launch Editor of *The Sunday Telegraph's* "Stella" magazine, now at *The Times* of London—she's unbeatable on how finally to make fashion your friend.

254

BIBLIOGRAPHY

p.17 M. Angelou, *I Know Why the Caged Bird Sings*, London, Virago Press. **p.157** M. Angelou, "Phenomenal Woman," *And Still I Rise*, London, Little, Brown Book Group Limited, 1986. **p.133** The Business of Fashion and McKinsey & Company, *The State of Fashion 2018*, 2017. **p.190** A. Cuddy, *Your Body Language May Shape Who You Are*, TEDGlobal 2012, 2012. www.ted.com/talks/amy_cuddy_your_body_language_shapes_who_you_are **p.13** E. Ferrante, Neopolitain Novels, New York, NY, Europa Editions. **p.180** M. Gladwell, *Blink: The Power of Thinking without Thinking*, London, Penguin Books Limited, 2006. **p.76** R. Lehmann, *Invitation to the Waltz*, London, Little, Brown Book Group Limited, 2006. **p.218** N. Mitford, *Love in a Cold Climate*, London, Penguin Books Limited, 2000. **p.24** E. Salter, *The Last Years of a Rebel: A Memoir of Edith Sitwell*, London, Bodley Head. **p.13** M. Twain, "The Czar's Soliloquy," *The North American Review*, Vol. 180, no. 580 (Mar., 1905), pp.321-326. **p.152** T. Wolfe, *The Bonfire of the Vanities*, London, Vintage, Random House, 2010. **p.180** V. Woolf, *Orlando: A Biography*, London, Vintage, Penguin Random House, 2016.